The Palgrave Lacan Series

Series Editors
Calum Neill
Edinburgh Napier University
Edinburgh, UK

Derek Hook
Duquesne University
Pittsburgh, USA

Jacques Lacan is one of the most important and influential thinkers of the 20th century. The reach of this influence continues to grow as we settle into the 21st century, the resonance of Lacan's thought arguably only beginning now to be properly felt, both in terms of its application to clinical matters and in its application to a range of human activities and interests. The Palgrave Lacan Series is a book series for the best new writing in the Lacanian field, giving voice to the leading writers of a new generation of Lacanian thought. The series will comprise original monographs and thematic, multi-authored collections. The books in the series will explore aspects of Lacan's theory from new perspectives and with original insights. There will be books focused on particular areas of or issues in clinical work. There will be books focused on applying Lacanian theory to areas and issues beyond the clinic, to matters of society, politics, the arts and culture. Each book, whatever its particular concern, will work to expand our understanding of Lacan's theory and its value in the 21st century.

Jessica L. Davis

Reading Foucault Through Lacan

From Hysteric to Analyst

palgrave
macmillan

Jessica L. Davis
Philosophy
American University of Sharjah
Sharjah, United Arab Emirates

ISSN 2946-4196 ISSN 2946-420X (electronic)
The Palgrave Lacan Series
ISBN 978-3-031-69737-1 ISBN 978-3-031-69738-8 (eBook)
https://doi.org/10.1007/978-3-031-69738-8

This Palgrave Macmillan imprint is published by the registered company Springer Nature Switzerland AG.
The registered company address is: Gewerbestrasse 11, 6330 Cham, Switzerland

Contents

Abbreviations

Michel Foucault

AK	The Archaeology of Knowledge
AME	Aesthetics, Method, Epistemology
BB	The Birth of Biopolitics
CT	The Courage of Truth
DÉ	Dits et Écrits, Tome 1
DÉ4	Dits et Écrits, Tome 4
DP	Discipline and Punish
EST	Ethics, Subjectivity and Truth
FS	Fearless Speech
GSO	The Government of Self and Others
HoS	The Hermeneutics of the Subject
HS1	The History of Sexuality, Volume 1
HS2	The History of Sexuality, Volume 2
IKA	Introduction to Kant's Anthropology
LCMP	Language, Counter-Memory, Practice
LWTK	Lectures on the Will to Know
MC	Madness and Civilization
MIP	Mental Illness and Psychology
NGH	Nietzsche, Genealogy, History
OD	The Order of Discourse
OT	The Order of Things

PK	Power/Knowledge
PPC	Politics, Philosophy and Culture
PP	Psychiatric Power
PS	The Punitive Society
PT	A Preface to Transgression
SMD	Society Must Be Defended
SP	The Subject and Power
TJF	Truth and Juridical Forms
TS	Technologies of the Self

Jacques Lacan

É	Écrits
ÉS	Écrits: A Selection
KS	Kant avec Sade
MT	My Teaching
PU	The Position of the Unconscious
SSD	The Subversion of the Subject and the Dialectic of Desire in the Freudian Unconscious
T	Television
SI	The Seminar of Jacques Lacan, Book I: Freud's Papers on Technique
SII	The Ego in Freud's Theory and in the Technique of Psychoanalysis
SIII	The Psychoses
SVII	The Ethics of Psychoanalysis
SVIII	Transference
SXI	The Four Fundamental Concepts of Psychoanalysis
SXVII	The Other Side of Psychoanalysis
SXX	Encore

List of Figures

1

Introduction—The Subversion of Intellect

> What I have said here is not 'what I think' but often rather what I wonder whether one couldn't think. (Foucault)

> I am not whenever I am the plaything of my thought; I think of what I am where I do not think to think. (Lacan)

The relationship between Jacques Lacan, the psychoanalyst, and Michel Foucault, the historian, is notoriously difficult to pin down. Formed by the different generations of the twenty-odd years that separated them, the two thinkers held disparate and often opposing views. The predominant reception of Lacan and Foucault is unsurprisingly one of incompatibility, if not hostility. It would be imprudent to suggest that the present book makes a definitive attempt to settle such disputes. Instead, it responds to a need to move beyond existing interpretations in order to re-examine the Lacan-Foucault relation in view of the commonalities that underpin their intellectual projects. The approach I adopt is thus similar to the work of cartography in that it maps trajectories of convergence between two heterogeneous discourses in recent French thought that can be broadly grouped under the signifiers 'Lacanian' and 'Foucauldian'.

J. L. Davis, *Reading Foucault Through Lacan*, The Palgrave Lacan Series,
https://doi.org/10.1007/978-3-031-69738-8_1

Despite the differences that divided Foucault and Lacan, their projects were in fact much closer than their respective adherents might care to admit. Briefly stated, this proximity was the result of a shared desire to formulate a discourse that would decenter the Western conception of the subject while maintaining a critical engagement with the phenomenon of subjectivity as it is understood in post-Kantian traditions. In a tribute to Lacan after his death in 1981, Foucault recalls their common aim to liberate "everything that is hidden behind the apparently simple use of the pronoun 'I'" (*DÉ4* 204). The similarity between Foucault's treatment of discourse and a certain psychoanalytic approach to the question of the subject is the main heuristic motivation for this book; it is also the justification of my attempt to read Foucault in light of Lacan's formalization of the discourses of psychoanalysis.

If one considers the notion of discourse in the most general sense as the abstraction of any written or oral process of communication through which meaning is transmitted, then one has to grant that Foucault's own manner of dealing with discourse is–discursive. With his archaeological and genealogical methods of critique, Foucault revealed the historical conditions that make a particular mode of conceptualization possible while simultaneously uncovering the discursive and institutional strategies that contribute to the formation of subjects. Individuals, groups, and social classes do not, therefore, constitute the target of Foucault's critique for they are subjects, that is, discursive constructs. Instead of erecting new boundaries that delimit human nature, Foucault aimed his discourse at other discourses, not human beings. Foucault's approach to discourse is, in this sense, contiguous with Lacan's for whom "a signifier is that which represents a subject … not for another subject, but for another signifier" (*SXI* 180–81). The signifier serves to link an individual to other signifiers, not to another individual. The subject is therefore an effect of the realm of signifiers and the subject's reality is provided by a field of discourses.

For Lacan, as for Foucault, the question of the subject is fundamental to the whole problematic of our human relation to the world. This relation is made possible by the Symbolic order. With its system of signifiers, the Symbolic is a function of the order of language itself. Our existence as subjects is made possible by the Symbolic experience. Indeed, "the essential part of human experience", Lacan observes, "can be located at the level where the symbol arises"; it is the dimension that makes signification possible (*SII* 255–56). Lacan understands the subject as both a relay of the Symbolic and a support for it. The subject does not produce its own meaning; rather, "signification is a function of a certain language which is and isn't the language of the subject—he receives it ready-made" (*SII* 374). From a Lacanian point of view, the subject is not whole and meaningful, but divided and split from within; we do not say what we mean. For this reason, the question of the subject concerns the story of its own history precisely because this is kept hidden: as Lacan explains, "man's life is oriented by a problematic which is not that of life-experience, but that of destiny, that is to say the meaning of man's story/history"[1] (*SII* 58). This approach to the question of the subject is equally important for Foucault who endeavored to analyze our human failure to understand our own history and to show, in turn, how this affects human existence. To carry out this project, Foucault found it necessary:

> [T]o dispense with the constituent subject, to get rid of the subject itself, that is to say, arrive at an analysis which can account for the constitution of the subject within a historical framework. (*PK* 117)

It is this reflection on the centrality of discourse that is conspicuously absent in recent scholarship depicting the Foucault-Lacan relation. In her article titled "Biopolitics, Sexuality and the Unconscious", Alenka Zupančič (2016) focuses on a conceptual omission in volume I of *The History of Sexuality* where Foucault charges psychoanalysis with the potential to become, under certain conditions, another technology of modern power. For Zupančič, Foucault's failure to mention the unconscious is significant since the entire theory of repression—on which Foucault's theory of power implicitly depends—is decided by this concept. Foucault was not, however, primarily a theorist of power and even refuted this title on occasion. Rather, his writings sought to disrupt power mechanisms that obtain in Western societies by disclosing the contingency of truths that validate its discourses, that is, the circuit in which the

[1] The French word *histoire* can mean both "story" and "history," whence the meaningful ambiguity of the question.

subject finds itself integrated. In a certain regard, Foucault's approach to discourse is similar to that of Lacan's in that it shares a rebellious relationship to meaning which operates performatively at the level of the signifier and distances itself from the truth of philosophy. Although Zupančič is right to point out Foucault's capricious and, at times, hostile stance toward psychoanalysis, it is gratuitous to suggest that the manifest absence of the word 'unconscious' is tantamount to its disavowal. Ironically, this might be an occasion to heed Joan Copjec when she writes: "*don't read my words; read my desire!*".

Foucault, like Lacan, understood that if we are not bound to an image by an essence or a nature that subjects us to a sovereign cultural order, we are free to reinvest ourselves in a dependency on the Symbolic through which we might go beyond such images. In Lacanian theory, the subject forms an identity in the Imaginary but requires the Symbolic dimension to transcend this identity, which is felt to be an inadequate representation of the Real. If there is a visible and describable praxis to Foucault's writing, it can be understood as a commitment to this Symbolic opening which not only founds the subject's existence in relation to the discourse of the other, instead of Truth, but also communicates a desire to make manifest the unlimited human potential for re-fabricating meaning. The dissolution of subjective consciousness in Foucault's approach does not eliminate the subject *tout court*; the subject is still present in discourse as the presence of an absence, the subject as non-being. This produces a shift in perspective where thought is oriented toward the unconscious subject: "the unfolding of a space in which it is once more possible to think" (*OT* 342).

A further attempt to assert an irreducible difference between Lacan and Foucault was recently announced by Jean-Claude Milner in his book *A Search for Clarity*. Although Milner's commentary on Foucault occupies a peripheral concern relative to the question of how Lacan viewed the relationship between psychoanalysis and science, the third chapter develops a noteworthy discussion on the status history in each thinker's work. Whereas Lacan posits major historical breaks that affect all compossible discourses without immunity, Milner remarks that Foucault can only conceive of a system of independent and non-synchronous breaks by virtue of his methodological approach.[2] In the late 1960s, Lacan demonstrates a key instance of this break in the discursive passage from the Master to the University as illustrated in his formalization of the discourses on the *other side* of psychoanalysis. The emergence of psychoanalysis, as Milner observes, testifies to the fact that psychic life itself is not immune from such a break: there is a distinctly modern subject "regardless of whether one chooses to distinguish it from an ancient subjectivity or assumes this subjectivity is born with modernity itself" (2021: 49).

Viewing the constant decouplings and multiple turbulences of Foucault's histories through the singular lens of a minor break risks downplaying the major epistemological break that informs his discursive strategy. In the 1960s, Foucault traced the emergence of the figure of 'man' as an epistemological concept to the early nineteenth century. Understood as both an object of knowledge and a subject that knows, 'man's' knowledge of himself is determined by a circular process. It is constituted by the empirical experience of his existence; this experience, in turn, is broken down into the facts that make up the framework of his thinking about himself and provide an epistemological validation for scientific knowledge. In *The Order of Things* (1994 [1966]) Foucault describes this condition as the predicament of the "empirico-transcendental doublet"; a divided subject whose speech calls out to be decoded. Foucault's concern for the historical production of this split subject complements Lacanian theory in that it accounts for the ways in which power is suffused with subjectivity. The problem for Foucault is therefore not only an epistemological one. The status of the subject in Western discourse has been guaranteed by an anthropological bias that furnishes knowledge with a propensity for turning into a political instrument of subjection.

Just as Foucault's discourse does not do away with 'man', but only relocates the human outside the constraints of an anthropology, it does not so much discard the subject as it redefines the subjective function of 'man' in the context of discourse. No longer determined by

[2] As an example of the non-homology and non-coincidence of minor historical breaks in Foucault's work, Milner points out that Christianity constituted a break in sexuality, but not for madness.

anthropological transcendentalism, 'man' finds himself bound to the fate of humankind, to the determinisms of the Symbolic order—of what mediates between 'man' and others, between 'man' and his universe. Foucault's position in discourse thus refuses to provide an all-embracing perspective that reveals order and coherence; it finds instead only fragments—distinct segments determined by specific rules and according to the Symbolic economy in which they operate. By impelling thought toward the invisible yet ever-present determinisms of the Symbolic and disrupting the habitual tendency to provide discourse with the ontological guarantee of Imaginary subjects, Foucault's approach demands that we consider writing as an activity "that unfolds like a game that inevitably moves beyond its own rules and finally leaves them behind" in order to "create an opening where the writing subject endlessly disappears" (*LCMP* 116). In this respect, Foucault's discursive approach provides an apt illustration for the Lacanian aphorism: "I *am* there where I do not *think*" (*ÉS* 126).

My aim in this book is to read Foucault *through* Lacan. The general arc of my reading depends, first and foremost, on delineating the critical relation that Foucault's discourse maintains with traditional modes of intellection in order to underscore the fundamentally subversive thrust of his approach. The subversion I identify in Foucault's discourse is eminently positive: it is the negation of a negation. Foucault highlighted areas of knowledge inspired by a positivistic outlook and presented them as a negation, that is, effective at establishing areas of exclusion as well as privilege. What has been negated, from Foucault's perspective, is the dimension of human experience that is not amenable to conscious and rational control. It is here where I understand some of Lacan's theoretical schemas and concepts to be helpful in elucidating Foucault's critical strategy—a strategy that emphasizes a capacity for reorienting thought toward the function, effect, and uses of discourse. This book interprets the critical impetus of Foucault's approach from the perspective of Lacan's theorization of the four discourses.

Lacan defined discourse as a social link founded on language. In Seminar XVII: *The Other Side of Psychoanalysis* (1969–1970) (2007), Lacan proposed four fundamental discourses, the Master, the Analyst, the University, and the Hysteric, to represent the four possible formulations of the Symbolic network that social bonds can take. A distinctive feature of Lacan's theorization of discourse lies in its articulation of the relation between language (the Symbolic) and that which is not language (the Real). This allows Lacan to explain how a given discourse or text affects human subjects—both temporarily and consciously, as well as more permanently or structurally—, whether they are its producers or recipients (Bracher 1994). Like Foucault, Lacan develops a view of how subjects are shaped by discourse and yet retain a capacity for resistance. The purpose of Lacan's schema is to show what sort of changes are possible and how they might be brought about through permutations of a four-term configuration showing the relative positions—the agent, the other, the product, and truth—of four terms: the subject, the master signifier, knowledge and *petit a* (Fig. 1.1).

Each discourse stands in an inverted relation to the other, with the Master as the "other side" of the Analyst referred to in the title of Lacan's Seminar XVII, and the University as the inverse of the Hysteric. This structural inversion is an example of a central paradox that underlies Lacanian theory: the sexual impasse. As Slavoj Žižek notes, a key distinction between psychoanalysis and philosophy lies in their treatment of sexual difference: "for philosophy, the subject is not inherently sexualized, […] whereas psychoanalysis makes sexualization a kind of formal, a priori condition for the very emergence of the subject" (1998: 81). In Lacan's schema, the Master and the University represent 'masculine' discourses of power, each striving to establish a complete and closed social order. In contrast, the Hysteric and the Analyst are positioned as 'feminine' discourses of critique, engaged in the mediating effect of the Symbolic and adept at discerning various strategies of epistemological closure. This book examines the structure of Foucault's critique from the

S1	S2	a	$\$$	Master			
	S2	a	$\$$	S1	University		
		a	$\$$	S1	S2	Analytic	
			$\$$	S1	S2	a	Hysteric

Fig. 1.1 Series of elements and their permutations in the Four Discourses

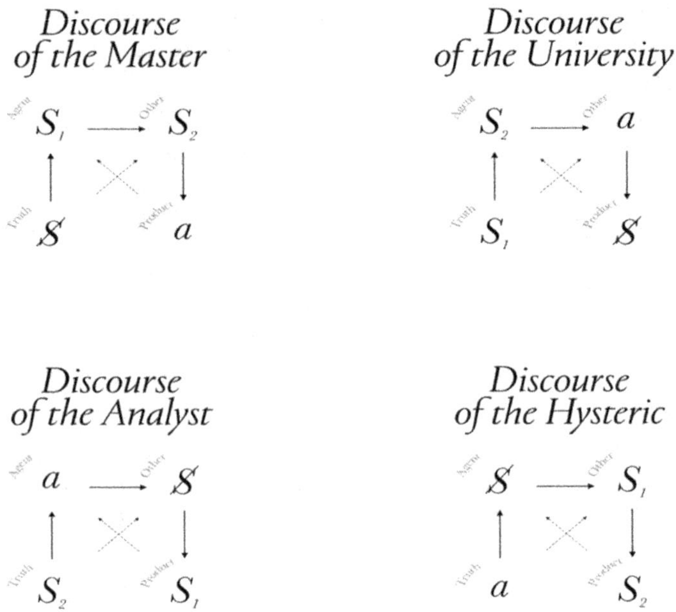

Fig. 1.2 The Four Discourses

point of view of the Hysteric and the Analyst, particularly in their opposition to the University and the Master (Fig. 1.2).

The act of reading and writing about Foucault in this manner leads me to impose an unwarranted unity on Foucault's oeuvre. My subject, however, is such that this tactic seems unavoidable. The insight stressed in this book is meant to present Foucault's critical project in its metonymical relationship with traditional modes of intellection and as an effective instrument of change. A preliminary point of departure for grasping the structure of Foucault's critique is through its connection to Immanuel Kant's critical philosophy. Foucault's interest in Kant spans his entire career. Many of his writings point to an opposition between two possible Kantian legacies: a transcendental legacy, to which Foucault refused to subscribe, that establishes universal rules of truth; on the other hand, a critical legacy, in which he situated himself, that challenges the present on the basis of a diagnosis of 'who we are'. While the former focuses on a formal inquiry into the conditions of possibility of true knowledge, the latter investigates the practices necessary for transforming ourselves to gain access to truth. The two Kantian traditions provide the basic coordinates for mapping Foucault's position of critique onto the Hysteric and the Analyst, respectively.

Divided into two parts, the organizational structure of the book follows from this split within Foucauldian critique. Foucault's critique of Kantian critique serves as a leitmotif for Part I, "The Hysteric's Discourse". From the standpoint of the hysteric subject, established knowledge—and the laws and politics derived from it—are symptomatic; they are inherently flawed and marked by a sense of inadequacy and loss. Chapters 2–4 cover the period from the early to mid-1970s in which Foucault conceives of critique along the anti-Kantian directives that Friedrich Nietzsche laid out in *On the Genealogy of Morals* (1881). One of Foucault's principal insights is an understanding of the intricate and deceitful ways in which discourse establishes knowledge and imposes truths. This insight pertains to the question of identity, but even more to the eminently political nature of discourse; it points to Foucault's involvement with particular kinds of struggles that revolve around the question 'who are we'. In Part I of the book, I conceptualize Foucault's historical approach to critique in terms of the problematic of a hysterical questioning directed at Kant's transcendental schema of knowledge that marked the division of the modern subject.

Chapter 2 "Hystorical Critique", introduces Foucault's lecture course "The Will to Know" (1971–1972) as a necessary supplement to his essay "Nietzsche, Genealogy, and History" (1971) in which he develops a problematic of genealogy centered on a particular epistemological predisposition. Highlighting the contrast Foucault establishes in his lecture course between two conflicting paradigms of the *will to know*, I present the Nietzschean model as an analysis of the 'de-implication' of knowledge and truth. This provides an interpretive frame for Foucault's provocative claim that "knowledge is not made for understanding; it is made for cutting" (*NGH* 154). When applied to historical critique, the concept of 'de-implication' brings into focus an elided reality of Western discourse by placing a maximal distance between subject and object. Drawing on Gérard Wajcman's (2003) account of the riddle of hysteria, I show how the hysteric subject embodies this structural division—and thus the violence inherent in all discourse— through a castrating game that systematically subverts existing modes of explanation and rationalization. Chapter 2 conceptualizes the epistemological thrust of Foucault's genealogical critique from the perspective of the Hysteric's discourse.

Chapter 3, "The Body's Refusal", combines a precise explication of Lacan's theory of the four discourses with an account of how Foucault's genealogy of knowledge operates within this schema, anchored around the Hysteric's discourse. Building on Lacan's concept of discourse as an 'apparatus of *jouissance*' and his view of the body as an 'enjoying substance', I examine how genealogy enables a materialist historiography that exposes power's violent effects on the body. In the corpus of Foucault's genealogies, bodies are acted upon in discursively constituted institutional settings where resistances are rarely constructed, and struggles are not engaged. I introduce Foucault's lecture course "Psychiatric Power" (1973–1974), particularly his analysis of the "great maneuvers of hysteria", as providing a crucial counterexample. Chapter 3 establishes a metaphorical parallel between the "insurrection of hysterics" in the late nineteenth century and Foucault's "insurrection of subjugated knowledges" in the twentieth century, to explain how the "body" and "agency" interact in a genealogical framework. From the standpoint of the hysteric subject, I demonstrate that resistance is enacted through the body's refusal to comply with the scientific administrative inquisition that determines the subject's identity.

Chapter 4, "Foucault's Theatre of War", presents the thematic of constant war as a logical framework for grasping the genealogical use of history which has the potential to bring about its own wreckage with telling political underpinnings. The auto-destructive structure of Foucault's hystorical critique locates a point of impossibility for its own operations which I approach from Lacan's account of the Real as the impossible qua discursive formalization. Drawing on clinical perspectives, I explain how Foucault's genealogical staging of "repeated scenes of violence" brings into focus the binary structure of the modern discursive arena as an ongoing struggle between the psychoanalytic 'forces' of hysterical desire (the Hysteric) and perverse drive (the University). The structural impasse of the Real in Foucault's hystorical critique leads to a comment on the topological structure of the Möbius band in a discursive context. I conclude

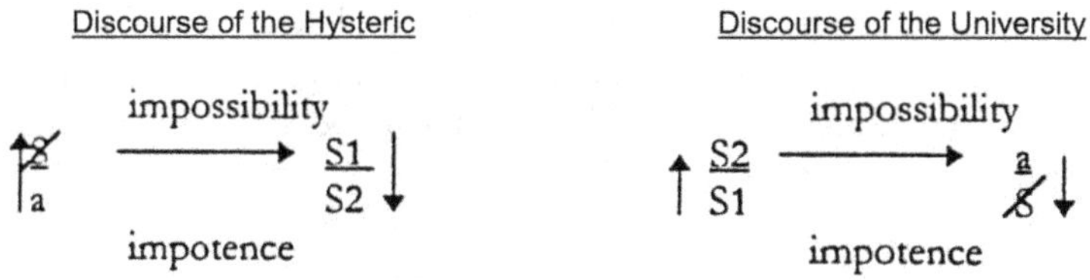

Fig. 1.3 The Discourses of the Hysteric and the University

Chap. 4 by arguing that the framework of war impels Foucauldian critique toward a moment outside of discourse and thus forces him to pass to another one (Fig. 1.3).

Part II, "The Analyst's Discourse", examines the discursive passage from Hysteric to Analyst in conjunction with Foucault's retrospective claim that his work aligns with Kant's critical legacy. From 1978 to 1984, Foucault began to redefine critique as an engagement with the present that demands a historico-practical test of limits. In a cluster of interviews, texts, and articles on Enlightenment, Foucault claims that Kant transformed the question of the present in such a manner that philosophy itself became the surface of emergence of its own discursive reality, capable of articulating its own meaning, value and singularity. The task of the modern philosopher, in Foucault's estimation, is to engage in a "critical ontology of ourselves in the present" (*PT* 127), which he understands as an attempt to confront the structural mastery of philosophy in a discursive context. Lacan, like Foucault, sees philosophical discourse as partaking in the discourse of mastery: "who can deny that philosophy has ever been anything other than a fascinating enterprise for the master's benefit?" (*SXVII* 23). Foucault's redefinition of critique decenters the position of the universal philosopher who acts as a master of truth in favor of the historically situated standpoint of the specific intellectual whose work is tied to a particular context. The latter can be described as an "analyst of the present" who takes on the task of understanding how and why "that-which-is might no longer be that-which-is" (*AME* 450). Foucault thus underscores a mode of historical critique in which human beings problematize their relation to the present in ways that usher possibilities for separation and transformation:

> it will not deduce from the form of what we are what it is impossible for us to do and to know; but it will separate out, from the contingency that has made us what we are, the possibility of no longer being, doing, or thinking what we are, do, or think. (*PT* 127)

The modern subject—and the Kantian critique that starts from it—are grounded in contingent historical conditions which thereby reveal the possibility for their transformation. Foucault's purpose is thus comparable to Lacan's, since it also consists in showing that "man is not an object, but a being in the process of realizing itself, something metaphysical" (*SII* 130). As a practitioner of the Symbolic function, the analyst aims to divest our Self from the privilege we derive from evidence that is nothing more than a historical happenstance, and to make us discover that our "syntax is linked to the dimension of the unconscious" (*SXI* 66). Foucault's writing has a similar effect: the truth of the subject finds itself displaced from an inner subjective certitude to the realm of a discourse that develops in historical contingency. Chapters 5–7 analyze Foucault's reconceptualization of Kantian critique from the perspective of the Discourse of the Analyst, in its opposition to the Discourse of the Master (Fig. 1.4).

Chapter 5, "*Le Point de Capiton:* Two Kantian Legacies", sketches Foucault's discursive passage from Hysteric to Analyst, drawing on the conceptual landscape that Lacan developed to give new rigor to the psychoanalytic account of language. Applying the Lacanian concept of the *point de capiton* (quilting point) and related notion of the 'signifying chain', I outline the retroactive logic of the determination of meaning as it figures in the act by which Foucault symbolizes his philosophical project of critique. I interpret Foucault's repeated attempts to situate himself

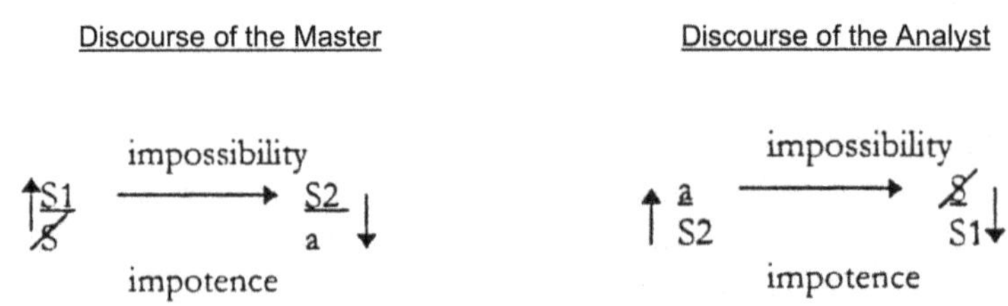

Fig. 1.4 The Discourses of the Master and the Analyst

in relation to the symbolic economy of Kant's critical philosophy as a key instance of 'the slippage of signification'. The identificatory signifier 'Kant' has a shifting and contingent signified in Foucault's discourse with no stable referent. Drawing on the elementary cell of Lacan's graph of desire, I present Foucault's lecture course "The Government of Self and Others (1982–1983)" (2010) as the site of chain's punctuation: the retroactive moment when the signifier and signified form an attachment. Chapter 5 offers an account of how Foucault's critical ontology symbolizes the contingent dimension of Kant's transcendental legacy and realizes the symbolic by situating the question of enlightenment in a past and future signifying relation to the Real.

Chapter 6, "The Parrhesiastic P(a)ct", charts the consideration on the part of both Foucault and Lacan of an ethic of the 'discursive act' to highlight the ethico-political stakes that inform their work. I identify 'freedom' in Foucault and 'polymorphous perversion' in Lacan as key factors that define the ontological precarity—the shifting and uncertain context—in which ethics emerges. I argue that Foucault and Lacan both formulate an account of ethics centered on the act of speaking which does not suppose the fixity or rigidity of identity as its ground. I distinguish an ethics of speaking from an ethics of coincidence with oneself or one of confession and self-disclosure. Drawing on Lacan's L schema, I explain how his concept of 'full speech' and later account of the ethic of the well-spoken (*bien-dire*) is correlated with the implication of the speaking subject in the enjoyment that her symptom denounces. The discursive context in which speech introduces a critical interruption that modifies the speaker's mode of being is equally explored in Foucault's analysis of the ancient practice of *parrhesia* in which the speaker uses their free courage to demonstrate reflexivity toward their own position of enunciation. Chapter 6 provides a picture of psychoanalytic praxis as an act that transpires inside the frame of speech and depends on the position of the Analyst to maintain that frame.

Chapter 7, "Towards a New Erotics", reflects on the juncture in which each thinker approaches the question of subjectivity not in terms of who we *must* be, but how we might live in the world without the supposition of a fundamental or unproblematic identity, or where it becomes the object of analysis. I examine erotic experience through the lens of an affective encounter, highlighting the Imaginary dimension in which the relationship between analyst and analysand unfolds in the analytic situation. Drawing on Seminar VIII: Transference (1960-61) I examine Lacan's claim that transference manifests as a love of knowledge, with the Analyst embodying the address for love through an engagement with the Real. Shifting the discussion to Foucault's analysis of Plato's Socratic dialogues, I consider two erotic domains ('care' and 'psychagogy') in which philosophy is understood not as a form of knowledge dependent on the Master's reason, but rather a certain style of discourse that aims at transforming both the speaker and the listener. Chapter 7 concludes with a reflection on my own subjective encounter with Lacan and Foucault as erotic thinkers and the way in which the eros of their thought can be linked to ethical experience.

References

Bracher, M. (1994) "On the Psychological and Social Functions of Language: Lacan's Theory of the Four Discourses", in M. Bracher, M. W. Alcorn Jr., R. J. Corthell, & F. Massardier-Kenney (eds.) *Lacanian Theory of Discourse: Subject, Structure and Society,* New York/London: New York University Press.

Copjec, J. (1994) *Read My Desire: Lacan Against the Historicists.* London: Verso.

Foucault, M. (1994) *The Order of Things.* Translated from the French by A. Sheridan. New York: Vintage Books.

———. (2010) The Government of Self and Others: Lectures at the Collège de France, 1982–1983, Gros, F. (ed.). Translated from the French by G. Burchell. New York: Palgrave Macmillan.

Lacan, J. (2007) *The Seminar of Jacques Lacan, Book XVII: The Other Side of Psychoanalysis, 1969–1970,* J. A. Miller (ed.). Translated from the French by R. Grigg. New York: W.W. Norton and Company.

Milner, J.C. (2021) *A Search for Clarity: Science and Philosophy in Lacan's Oeuvre.* Translated from the French by E. Pluth. Northwestern University Press.

Wajcman, G. (2003) "The Hysteric's Discourse", in Žižek, S. (ed.) *Jacques Lacan: Critical Evaluations in Cultural Theory. Vol 1: Psychoanalytic Theory and Practice*. New York: Routledge, pp. 186–198.

Zupančič, A. (2016) "Biopolitics, Sexuality and the Unconscious". Paragraph, 39(1), 49–64.

Žižek, S. (1998) "Four Discourses, Four Subjects", in Žižek, S. (ed.) *Cogito and the Unconscious*. Durham: University of Duke Press, pp. 74–113.

Part I

The Hysteric's Discourse

2

Hystorical Critique

2.1 Introduction

In his article "Nietzsche, Genealogy and History" (1971) Foucault makes two equally provocative yet ambiguous claims. The first concerns the historical examination of the notion of truth which, as Foucault argues, reveals that "all knowledge rests on injustice" and that "the instinct for knowledge is malicious (something murderous, opposed to the happiness of mankind)" (*NGH* 163). The second comes from Foucault's insistence on the distinction between traditional and "effective" history. Opposing the genealogist's relationship to knowledge to that of the historian, Foucault asserts that "knowledge is not made for understanding; it is made for cutting" (154). I argue that these claims formulate an explicit problematic of genealogy which allows us to grasp the epistemology driving Foucault's "hystorical critique".[1] To develop this point of view, I focus

[1] I present Chap. 2 as an exploration of "hystorical critique," linking Lacan's formalization of the Hysteric's discourse to Foucault's genealogical critique, described, via Nietzsche, as a passion for knowledge-*savoir*.

J. L. Davis, *Reading Foucault Through Lacan*, The Palgrave Lacan Series,
https://doi.org/10.1007/978-3-031-69738-8_2

mainly on Foucault's inaugural lecture course "The Will to Know" (1970–1971) to decode the decidedly Nietzschean lexis.[2]

Before the publication of "Nietzsche, Genealogy and History," Foucault devoted a series of lectures to Nietzsche first at the experimental Vincennes university in the winter of 1969–1970, then at New York State University at Buffalo in 1970, and after at McGill University at Montreal in 1971. Despite not being delivered in Paris, these last two lectures are included as part of the volume *Lectures on the Will to Know* (2013). The title of the course itself may indicate a point further back in time. In July 1967 Foucault wrote a letter in which he recognized "the morphology of the will to know in European civilization" as the reason Nietzsche had always fascinated him (*LWTK* 266).[3] During that year, Foucault identified and isolated a will to know (*savoir*) that cannot be assimilated into knowledge (*connaissance*) which would shape the trajectory of his future lectures. Speaking at the Collège de France in December 1970, Foucault avows that he could have given the title "The Will to Know" to most of the historical analyses carried out to that point and prompts his audience to view "all of these analyses—past or still to come—as fragments for a morphology of the will to know" (1).

One prevalent theme in post-war French thought was the enthusiastic reception of Nietzsche (and Heidegger) and the consequent rejection of metaphysics and Cartesian rationalism. In "The Will to Know" this theme is noticeably reflected in the opposition Foucault establishes between Aristotle (in the *Metaphysics*) and Nietzsche. According to Foucault, Nietzsche and Aristotle provide two extreme and opposing paths through which to analyze the western *will to know*. The Nietzschean route leads to the outside (or perhaps the underside) of knowledge. In Sect. 2.2.2, "The Outside of Knowing", I explain how the Nietzschean passion for knowledge, as defined by Foucault, discovers not an ontological foundation that can either liberate or repress, but an unconscious war among drives, a rivalry of instincts, a will to appropriation. This description not only resonates with the situation of post-war Europe, still

[2] Foucault's inaugural address at the Collège "The Order of Discourse" (1970) is not included as part of the volume *Lectures on the Will to Know*. In this chapter, I provide some references to this text.

[3] Michel Foucault, letter of 16 July 1967, *Dits et Écrits*, vol. I, p. 31; "Quarto" ed., vol. I, p. 41.

recoiling perhaps from images of mass annihilation, but it also serves as a profound castigation of the goal of metaphysics (or “first philosophy”) to discern being and the world.

The “outside” is a thematic that interested Foucault, earlier, in the mid-1960s. This is especially evident in his essay on the work of Maurice Blanchot titled “The Thought from Outside” (1966). In this text, Foucault describes western thought as being enclosed within certain codes and structures which have historically constituted and delineated it. Against the notion of a pure, interior space that could serve as the repository of all meaning, Foucault maintains that the task and responsibility of thought are to try to reflect the outside of these structures in which thinking has remained historically situated. This trenchant critique of interiority is arguably present in Foucault’s lecture course “The Will to Know”. In Sect. 2.2.1, “The Desire to Know”, I introduce the theoretical structure, outlined in Foucault’s presentation of Aristotle, in which desire, knowledge, and truth are enfolded in the same epistemological drive, thwarting the introduction of exteriority in philosophical discourse. Whence the importance, for Foucault, of the Nietzschean outside which refers not only to knowledge but also to the thought from outside the (metaphysical) discourse of philosophy.

Foucault’s essays on art and literature in the early 1960s share a similarity in their concerns which include, amongst other things, the relation of language to madness and death. In many of these writings, Foucault is less interested in the specificity of the literary as such and more concerned with how the works of literature could function paradigmatically as counter-discourses, or as indexes pointing towards an exit from dialectics. In “A Preface to Transgression” (1963), written as an homage to Georges Bataille, Foucault celebrates the way his work pushed against and transgressed the boundaries of language. In this text, Foucault also reflects on philosophy’s (in)ability to open up to madness. These two points offer a specific angle through which to grasp the significance of Nietzsche’s positioning contra Aristotle by Foucault in “The Will to Know”. In Sect. 2.3, “Madness in the Method”, I first consider the “genealogical aspect” of Foucault’s historical analysis which refers to the conditions of emergence and of the transgression of discourse *on both sides* of the boundary, I then define the form in which Nietzsche's madness can be shown to "speak" to philosophy.

Foucault's presentation of the Nietzschean system of knowledge (*savoir*) discloses the possibility for a historical analysis of "de-implication" which chisels a hole in Aristotle's theoretical structure and western philosophy more broadly. This involves a situation in which knowledge and truth are separated from their supposed original affiliation. Contrary to traditional epistemology, it also suggests a plurality of relations without a subject or object. Foucault thus highlights the event-like character of knowledge and truth which violently impose an order on an otherwise unknowable reality. The notion that the subject-object relation is not the foundation, but the product of knowledge provides recourse to another discourse. In Sect. 2.3.2, "The Riddle of Hysteria" I introduce Gerard Wajcman's presentation of the Hysteric's discourse as a means of apprehending the critical function of the term "de-implication" through a castrating game directed at the discourse of mastery. Crucially, I draw a connection between the historical analysis of "de-implication", from which Foucault derives and adapts his own method of genealogy, with the function of the riddle of hysteria in that both entail a certain "Hystoricization of Truth" (2.4) which enables us to think "knowledge as a historical process before any problematic of truth" (*LWTK* 214).

Chapter 2, therefore, marks a significant contribution to the literature on Foucault and Lacan in that it establishes an entry point for thinking Foucault's genealogical method through Lacan's formalization of the Hysteric's discourse which he presents in Seminar XVII: *The Other Side of Psychoanalysis* (1969–1970). To my knowledge, this is the first attempt to theorize the Discourse of the Hysteric within the framework of the epistemology driving Foucault's hystorical critique which I identify as the passion for knowledge-*savoir*. The theme of Chap. 2 inserts itself into two main groups of discussions and debates. The first concerns Foucault's "Nietzscheanism" which I approach in terms of the larger problematic of a hysteric(al) questioning of Kant's transcendent schema of knowledge. The second, related to the first, concerns the critiques of Foucault's historicism from psychoanalytic theorists. One extreme example comes from Joan Copjec (1994) who argues that historicism wants nothing to do with desire. The implicit aim of Chap. 2, with its emphasis on the

Hysteric's discourse and the genealogist's passion for knowledge-*savoir*, is to reinvigorate the debate around the question: where is Foucault in relation to desire in the early to mid-1970s?

2.2 Nietzsche Contra Aristotle

In this section, I consider the distinction that Foucault draws in his lecture course "The Will to Know" (1970–1971) between a Nietzschean and Aristotelian paradigm for truth. Foucault dedicates his first course at the Collège de France to investigating the origins of the *will to know* in the western philosophical tradition. This inquiry begins with a basic acknowledgment of the direct and seemingly unproblematic relationship between will and knowledge and knowledge and truth. Foucault questions both the strategic function of the argument that posits a natural and undisputed tendency toward knowledge in every human being as well as the implications of truth's portrayal as free from connections of power. From the outset of the course, Foucault states that the game he would like to play will involve seeing:

> [W]hether the *will to truth* is not as profoundly historical as any other system of exclusion; whether it is not as arbitrary in its roots as they are; whether it is not as modifiable as they are in the course of history; whether like them it is not dependent upon and constantly reactivated by a whole institutional network; and whether it does not form a system of constraint which is exercised not only on other discourses but on a whole series of other practices. In short, it is a matter of seeing what real struggles and relations of domination are involved in the *will to truth*. (*LWTK*2, my emphasis)

Daniel Defert remarks that Foucault's course is inaugural in more than one sense; it bears "recognition of the speaker's new status" as chair of the history of systems of thought and "marks his entry into the ancient beginnings of philosophy", even though the doxa only associates his later work with Greek Antiquity (2013: 262). Inaugural, too, is Foucault's recycling of the mode of reasoning used in the *History of the Madness* (1961) for the history of philosophy. Parallel to the book, Foucault's course uncovers an original gesture that led to a violent act of social exclusion. Only this time the division that interests Foucault is not that of madness and reason, but truth and falsehood. As signaled previously in "The Order of Discourse" (1970), Foucault suspects that the opposition of true and false constitutes a system of exclusion of its own, one that grows "stronger, deeper, and more implacable" than the traditional schemas of the prohibition of speech and the rejection of madness (*OD* 56).

Foucault raises the question of truth in the history of philosophy in a particular way. Rather than inserting its events into a single interpretive scheme that one would need to surpass or overcome, Foucault historicizes philosophy by locating the external events that caused it to rethink itself. The lectures situate the historical division between truth and falsity at the time between Plato and Hesiod, a period which saw the banishing of the Sophist and sophistic truth from philosophical discourse. Foucault considers this act of exclusion to be a watershed moment in the history of western thought, claiming that it is here that: "truth was displaced from the ritualized, efficacious and just act of enunciation, towards the utterance itself" (*OD* 54). The narrowing of the gap between thought and speech gave rise to new principles of restraint that subjected true discourse to an order, cutting off its link to the exercise of power. In response, Foucault proposes a kind of genealogy of philosophical speech starting from the inception of its systematization in ancient Greece to identify the tactics and strategies through which philosophy has tried, throughout history, to connect will, knowledge, and truth.

The lectures also mark Foucault's attempt to cast aside traditional notions of the passion for truth and knowledge. In their place, Foucault draws a contrast between an Aristotelian conception of the "pleasure in theoretical contemplation" supposed to be natural to every human being, and a Nietzschean conception of the *will to know* (*LWTK* 12). The "will" in question is neither contemplative nor natural, nor everywhere the same. With Nietzsche, Foucault insists that knowledge is seen as an "invention" and as an "event, or at least a series of events" (227). Against the regime of speech installed by Aristotle which takes for granted the natural human disposition toward knowledge, the model of knowledge supplied by Nietzsche is fundamentally "interested". The "interest" of knowledge involves a basic and paradoxical "falsification" which allows people to say the truth about some things but not about others (227). It was, at the time, these features of the *will to know* that Foucault sought to develop in his historical analyses of "discursive practices" which show how knowledge is produced in contingent and plural practices across different sites.[4] What is less obvious and thus open for further reflection is the mode of speech (re)introduced by Nietzsche.

It is against this backdrop that Foucault's lecture course "The Will to Know" assumes critical importance. If the theme of the course is to examine "what real struggles and relations of domination are involved in our *will to truth*" as noted in the quotation above, then Foucault must make a methodological decision. Should the choice of truth over falsity be studied on its own historical terms or as part of a morphology of the *will to know*?[5] By raising this question Foucault situates truth in relation to a further layer of analysis between knowledge-*connaissance* and knowledge-*savoir*.[6] Due to the inadequacy of historical instruments provided by epistemology, Foucault argues that historians of science have traditionally neglected the discursive events that have led to the question of the *will to know*. In an attempt to fill the lacuna, the two paradigms that Foucault surveys in the course, which were selected for their extreme and opposing forms, position Nietzsche contra Aristotle and correspond to the distinction between knowledge-*savoir* and knowledge-*connaissance*, respectively.

---

[4] For a further discussion of "discursive practices", see the summary Foucault gives of his 1970–1971 course under the title "History of Systems of Thought" in *Language, Counter-Memory and Practice*, pp. 199–201.

[5] In his review of the course, Juan Javier Rivera Andía (2015) distributes the lectures into two different groups. The first group traces the emergence of the *will to truth* along with its strong links to political and social transformations in ancient Greece. The second group, which constitutes the focus of the present chapter, centers on the unpacking of the two theoretical models of the *will to know*. Andía's review is available at: https://doi.org/10.4000/lectures.18113. [Accessed February 2019.]

[6] Foucault's use of the terms "*connaissance*" and "*savoir*" refers to the subject-object relation that is bilaterally constitutive of traditional epistemology. *Connaissance* designates the particular knowledge of various objects. Within each body of knowledge, the development of knowledge of objects coincides with the constitution of specific types of subjects. The process of simultaneously constituting the particular type of subject that is created in producing a particular *connaissance* is an instance of *savoir*. For a further overview of this distinction see Mary Beth Mader's (2014) entry on "Knowledge" in *The Cambridge Foucault Lexicon*, pp. 226–235.

2.2.1 The Desire to Know

In this section, I outline Foucault's presentation of the Aristotelian model of the *will to know* under the heading "The Desire to Know" which he analyses primarily on the basis of the *Metaphysics*.[7] In an attempt to situate its place in the history of systems of thought, Foucault claims that Aristotle's text is open to an external reading in which "we can identify an operation concerning philosophical discourse as it has existed in our civilization" (*LWTK* 5). Foucault summarizes two key operations that characterize the Aristotelian model in its capacity to act on the discourse of philosophy: (1) the re-introduction of knowledge beneath desire, and (2) the introduction of truth as the third element between desire and knowledge. I provide a sketch of the two operations and their consequences in the following paragraphs.

Beginning with Book I (A) of the *Metaphysics*, Foucault focuses his attention on the incipit: "all men by nature desire to know; the proof of this is the pleasure caused by sensations, for even apart from their usefulness, we enjoy them for themselves" (*LWTK* 5). This passage, according to Foucault, is vital to understanding some of the unquestioned assumptions of the western philosophical tradition. With these lines, Aristotle posits a *desire to know*, the universality or innate presence of desire in every human being, and its naturalness.

Foucault observes that Aristotle's argument implies three moves "that maybe cannot be completely superimposed on the move that allows one to descend quite simply from the general to the particular" (7). The move from knowledge to sensation is followed by the move which links the natural *desire to know* to the pleasure of sensation "in itself". Foucault highlights the third move from desire to the pleasure of "theoretical contemplation" to show how Aristotle aimed to establish continuity between the simple pleasure of sensation and what he considered the noblest and most complete form of knowledge, e.g., philosophy (13). It is here that Foucault identifies the first operation as "the reintroduction of knowledge under desire" on the basis of which desire could unfold (23). Foucault thus argues that the Aristotelian system is founded on the

[7] Minor references are given to the *Nicomachean Ethics* and *De Anima*.

"precondition of knowledge with regard to itself" in which desire, supposed to be prior to knowledge, is enveloped in knowledge from the start (15).

The envelopment of desire further suggests that the one who desires knowledge is also already "the one who possesses it or is capable of possessing it" (16). A subject can go from the *desire to know* (*savoir*) to knowledge (*connaissance*) simply by actualizing their nature. The implication is that knowledge (*savoir*) and desire do not appear "in two different places, possessed by two subjects or two powers", but are instead lodged in the same agency (16). This entails the absence of "violence, appropriation, and struggle" (16). Foucault locates in the Aristotelian system of knowledge-*connaissance* a prior unity, "mutual belonging" and "co-naturalness" between desire and knowledge insofar as the *desire to know* cannot want knowledge "for something other than itself because it is starting from knowledge that it wishes to know" (17). By the same token, this has the effect of protecting knowledge "from the exteriority and violence of desire" (16). The problem, as Foucault presents it, is that Aristotle appears to prescribe and define a certain "interiority" of philosophical discourse wherein:

> The *desire to know* is no more than a game of knowledge in relation to itself, it does no more than show its genesis, delay, and movement; desire is knowledge deferred, but made visible in the impatience of the suspense in which it is held. (38)

Foucault signals the inaccessibility of philosophy from the outside: desire, along with its transgressive dimensions, is presented as the outside in the theory of knowledge (38).[8] Furthermore, Foucault argues that the elimination of exteriority had the effect of tying philosophy and truth together in a certain mode. In his reading of the *Metaphysics*, Foucault underscores the extent to which the Aristotelian model of knowledge must assume the existence of truth and its specific role in ensuring the passage from desire to knowledge. The second operation put forth by the

---

[8] Alongside desire, Foucault states that the Sophist represents the outside in the history of philosophy.

Metaphysics is "the interplay of truth in relation to desire and knowledge" which constitutes the focal point of its systematicity (*LWTK* 24). Antonio Moretti observes that truth plays a key role because it ensures "the identity and unity of the subject" along with "the permanence, the stability of the object –which lies idle, waiting to be found" (2021, 137). For Foucault, truth functions as "the guarantee and foundation" of Aristotle's model; it founds the superiority of knowledge over desire and gives rise to the identity of the subject in desire and knowledge which have the same relationship to truth (24).

At stake in the Aristotelian system and western philosophy at large, argues Foucault, is the inability of will and desire to rid themselves of their subordination to knowledge (*connaissance*). This is due to their subjection to a fundamental relationship of truth; a truth, moreover, which is taken to be free from any connections of power. There is, within this schema, as Moretti suggests, "the perpetuation of the myth of the *uselessness* and *powerlessness* of truth" (2021, 137). What Foucault intends to render suspect is the original link presupposed by Aristotle between knowledge and truth which all subsequent philosophies maintained … until Nietzsche.

2.2.2 The Outside of Knowing

In this section, I introduce Foucault's presentation of the Nietzschean model of the *will to know* under the heading "The Outside of Knowing" which he analyzes primarily on the basis of texts from *The Gay Science* (1883), *Beyond Good and Evil* (1886), and *On Truth and Lies in a Nonmoral Sense* (1873). Foucault describes Nietzsche's role in the history of systems of thought as being "the first to release the *desire to know* from the sovereignty of knowledge (*connaissance*)" (*LWTK* 5). Foucault's presentation of the Nietzschean paradigm follows an inverted movement, reversing the two key operations highlighted in the Aristotelian model. In the following paragraphs, I provide a brief sketch of how Nietzsche disrupts the systematicity that underpins the theoretical structure of knowledge-desire-truth in Aristotle's model.

Foucault considers Nietzsche's claim in *The Gay Science* that behind knowledge lies something foreign, opaque, and irreducible: the "wall of non-knowledge" (*LWTK* 203). Knowledge, according to Nietzsche, arises from the interplay of instincts, impulses, desires and fear. In this model, desire is fundamental to knowledge but lacks any inherent connection to ends, origin, or nature. Foucault builds on this view in reference to Nietzsche's idea that knowledge is an invention (*Erfindung*), not something intrinsic to human nature. The absence of an innate knowledge instinct is demonstrated by the fact that "the intellect is at the service various instincts" (*LWTK* 203). Knowledge does not result from the harmony of these instincts; rather, it emerges from their conflict. By separating knowledge from the pleasure of pure contemplation, Nietzsche links it to the struggle of instincts and competing interests, which provide knowledge with a permanent and necessary support.

Guided by the rule of will, the Nietzschean model shows that knowledge is servile and dependent on "what is liable to interest the instincts that dominate it" (*LWTK* 227). Nietzsche understood interest to be radically prior to knowledge. For knowledge to arise, various impulses must first express their partial account of an object or event. Due to their differing and often opposing stances, conflicts might arise after which point a mutual pact can form, thus allowing, in turn, the impulses to watch over reason. In place of the certainty and affirmation that come from reason and experience, the rivalry of instincts produces doubt, negation, dissolution, and temporization. Foucault points here to the complex operation at stake in the invention of knowledge to underscore Nietzsche's provocative claim that desire and will exist outside of it.[9] Rather than grounding the act of knowing in a pre-existing, essential relationship to itself, Nietzsche situated the basis of knowledge in the interplay of differences.

The notion of a fundamentally interested knowledge produced as an event of the will is set in sharp contrast to the theoretical postulates advanced by Aristotle in the *Metaphysics.* For Nietzsche, knowledge is what rests on a network of relations that are "different in their form" and "in their points of support" (*LTWK* 210). Among them, a group of

[9] Foucault recognizes Freud, Nietzsche's counterpart, as someone who extended this scandal, p. 17.

relations are characterized by the fact that "they forcibly join together several differences" and impose the violence of a common mark (211). Foucault stresses this point in order to demonstrate that the subject-object relation is not the foundation of knowledge but is produced or rather invented by it. Nietzsche's model of the will to know accounts for knowledge by placing a maximal distance between subject and object, making them by-products that are far removed from each other. For Foucault, this represents a major deviation from all other philosophies "that have founded knowledge on a pre-established relation of subject and object, their sole concern being to bring them closer together, whether in a minimal form of sensation, or a pure consciousness (*cogito*), or a pure tautology (A = A)" (*LWTK* 212).

In his attempt to transcend the bounds of knowledge, Foucault observes that Nietzsche's discourse is susceptible to a Kantian objection: "either what we say about knowledge is true, but this can only be from within knowledge, or we speak outside of knowledge, but then nothing allows us to assert that what we say is true" (*LWTK* 26). According to Foucault, the only way out of this dilemma is to negate the co-implication of knowledge and truth. It is, therefore, through a reinterpretation of the relationship between knowledge, truth, and will that Foucault endeavors to assign Nietzsche a new place in the history of systems of thought. Unlike Heidegger who positioned Nietzsche within the tradition of metaphysics, tracinga continuous line from Aristotle through Descartes to Kant, Foucault situates him on a different path.[10] Foucault's approach reveals "the analysis of the de-implication of knowledge and truth" by which Nietzsche inaugurated a radical critique of the cultural and historical consequences of the Aristotelian paradigm:

> I think all the Nietzschean analysis of the desire, instinct, and *will to know*, irreducible to knowledge itself, is doubled by the work that makes it possible to de-implicate truth and knowledge; just as the Aristotelian reduction of the desire to know to knowledge recounted, in the background, the alliance of knowledge and truth. (*LWTK* 27)

[10] For a discussion on the differences between Foucault's and Heidegger's approach to Nietzsche, see Daniel Defert's commentary under the heading "A Nietzschean Greece" in the "Course Context", pp. 275–278.

In the absence of any natural link between truth, will, and knowledge, Foucault claims that the western philosophical tradition prefers to define their connection in terms of a mutual articulation through freedom: "the will must be free in order to give access to truth" (*LWTK* 215). For Nietzsche, this is an illusion; it implies the powerlessness of truth which sets aside its specific interests. It is also a particular kind of "falsification" which allows humans to cope in an otherwise unknowable world.[11] In contrast to the comforting image of appearances, Nietzsche sets "the murderous relentlessness of knowledge" against the welcoming mildness of a phenomenon (206). Instead of freedom, Nietzsche positions violence, compulsion, and domination as the pivotal point between truth and will. For Nietzsche, in other words, there is no natural desire to know. Truth and knowledge emerge as the outcome of specific historical-political conflicts which aim to dominate and prevail. Foucault argues that Nietzsche's model offers an analytic means by which to "extract knowledge-*savoir* from the interiority of knowledge-*connaissance* in order to rediscover in it the object of a willing, the end of a desire, the instrument of domination" (*LWTK* 17).

Through Nietzsche Foucault observes that the passion for knowledge is allied with "malice, mockery, contempt, [and] hatred" (*LWTK* 205). Behind the very act of knowledge is a war amongst the drives analogous to the struggle for supremacy amongst warriors. If knowledge is an invention, Foucault claims that is an even later invention. The notion of truth as the consequence of agonistic forces vying for their portion of reality highlights its event-like character. This approach to truth, as Moretti points out, makes it possible to put forth a history of knowledge that, "far from being a progressive unveiling of a *telos* or the search for a long-lost origin, is a history of the production of truth in actual struggles among the forces that attempt to seize it" (2021, 139). Crucially, Foucault's presentation of Nietzsche's model of knowledge and truth introduces the possibility of historical analysis as genealogy.

---

[11] Foucault cites a passage from *The Gay Science* in which Nietzsche claims that: "the character of the world is rather that of an eternal chaos", p. 204.

2.3 Madness in the Method

Before his appointment at the Collège de France in 1970, Foucault wrote *The Archaeology of Knowledge* (1969) in which he argued that knowledge (*savoir*) is neither identified with a cognitive faculty as in philosophical theory nor with science. The territory of discursive formations (knowledge) allowed Foucault to describe "epistemes" without having to resort to the divisions between truth and falsity, or science and ideology.[12] Foucault's title as chair of the history of "systems of thought" (epistemes) further solidified the orientation of his teachings vis-à-vis the other Collège chair, held by Jules Vuillemin, in the "philosophy of knowledge" (*connaissance*). As indicated in "The Order of Discourse", Foucault's position at the Collège coincided with a methodological shift of emphasis. Whereas the *Archaeology* analyzed discourse on its own terms, that is, without specific attention to relations of force, the genealogical aspect of his future analyses would study the conditions of emergence and of the transgression of discourse "on both sides of the boundary at once" (*OD* 71).

In this section, I consider Foucault's method of genealogy through the lens of madness. In particular, I argue that the lectures on "The Will to Know" establish a crucial albeit unexpected interface between philosophy and madness. In his earlier historical analyses, Foucault develops the view that madness is not a natural or unchanging thing but depends rather on the society in which it exists. This perspective is evident in the *History of Madness* (1961), a text in which Foucault addresses the question of philosophy's ability to open up to madness by looking at the work of artists and authors who went mad (e.g., Antonin Artaud, Van Gogh, and Nietzsche). It is in relation to the latter that Foucault casts madness as the

[12] At that time, Foucault's use of episteme was meant to designate a general framework of rules that operate beneath conscious processes, and which define a conceptual system of possibility that determines the limits of possible statements within a given epoch and domain.

"absence", "destruction", and "rupture" of an oeuvre.[13] Commenting on this bold and enigmatic statement, Angelos Evangelou stresses the way that Foucault challenges the concept of an oeuvre "by challenging its unity and its contribution to the authority of the author" (2017, 176).[14] This perspective raises important questions regarding the role of madness and the extent to which it might resist the methodology and implications of an autobiographical philosophy in ways that speak to Foucault's tastes for having no *face*.[15]

Another text in which Foucault addresses philosophy's (in)ability to open up to madness is "A Preface to Transgression", published in the "Hommage à Georges Bataille" issue of *Critique* one year after Bataille's death in 1963.[16] In this text, Foucault discusses the experience of the philosopher and the constitution of a language in which madness and philosophy come together at the juncture of what he calls "the play of transgression" (*PT* 42). Transgression, as Foucault understands it, refers to the category of "non-positive affirmation": an affirmation characterized by the lack of positivity at the center of its questioning, aware that it affirms nothing but the play of limit and of limitlessness (*PT* 36).[17] Foucault locates this category of philosophy in Nietzsche whom he opposes to Kant. Despite opening the space for western thought to reflect on the limits of reason in the *Critique of Pure Reason* (1781), Foucault criticizes Kant's *Anthropology* (1798) for having closed it and for sending human beings into a "confused sleep" from which Nietzsche awakens us with:

---

[13] Foucault first discusses this idea in the final pages of *History of Madness,* in the chapter "The Anthropological Circle" and, in more detail, in the essay which appeared three years after *History of Madness* and is attached as an Appendix to the 1972 edition of *History of Madness,* entitled "Madness, the Absence of an Œuvre".

[14] See Evangelou's recent text, *Philosophizing Madness from Nietzsche to Derrida* (2017).

[15] Foucault's preference for anonymity can be traced back to his lecture "What is an Author?" given at the Société Française de Philosophie on 22 February 1969. In the *Archaeology of Knowledge* (1972), published the same year, Foucault writes: "Do not ask who I am and do not ask me to remain the same. More than one person, doubtless like me, writes in order to have no face", p. 17.

[16] Established by Georges Bataille in 1946, *Critique* was a literary and philosophical journal reviewing publications in the human sciences.

[17] Foucault connects the notion of nonpositive affirmation with Blanchot's principle of contestation which he discusses in his study of Blanchot, "The Thought from Outside" published in *Critique* in 1966.

> [His] figures of tragedy, of Dionysus, of the death of God, of the philosopher's hammer, of the *Übermensch* approaching with the steps of a dove, of the Return. (*PT* 38)[18]

It is here that Foucault posits the construction of the "mad philosopher" by which he means "the experience of the philosopher who finds, not outside his language [...] but at the inner core of its possibilities the transgression of his philosophical being" (*PT* 42). Celebrating Bataille's erotic language which repeatedly "breaks down at the center of its space", Foucault holds that transgressive thought depends on the persistence to go to "[the] limit where the existence of language becomes problematic" and where philosophical subjectivity falls apart (*PT* 40). In search of a structural connection between madness and philosophy, Foucault's early writings privilege the space of art and literature for capturing the poetic experiences of the mad.[19] Similarly, John Caputo remarks that Foucault's belief in the "truth" of madness has nothing to do with "truth" in philosophy; rather, he "wants to hear what one says who has been driven to *extremis*" (2004, 119). Elaborating further, Caputo states:

> Foucault is not saying that the mad are the true philosophers but rather that they are precisely not philosophers at all, that they are the most forceful testimony to the breakdown of philosophy. They speak not with philosophical knowledge but with tragic knowledge. They have broken through the veil that philosophy lays over reality [...]. The mad speak *de profundis*, from the depths of an experience in which both the reassuring structures of ordinary life and the comforting reassurances of scientific or philosophical knowledge have collapsed. They experience the radical groundlessness of the world, the contingency of its constructs, both social and epistemic; [...] they are voices from an abyss. (2004, 120)

Through the distinction between the mad, on one hand, and the philosopher, on the other, Caputo's commentary allows us to highlight the

---

[18] For a detailed account of Foucault's criticism of Kant, see his *Introduction to Kant's Anthropology* (2008).

[19] Foucault's "early" writings refer here to *Mental Illness and Psychology* (1954) and the *History of Madness* (1961).

function of "tragic knowledge" in its ability to "speak" critically to philosophical knowledge. Before the enigma of a world was given by primitive forms of revelation, madness was seen as opening to the secrets of a Symbolic dimension. In the *Lectures on the Will to Know*, Foucault connects "tragic knowledge" to "knowledge-*savoir*" and, by extension, to the analysis of "de-implication" which makes possible historical critique as genealogy (*LWTK* 16). In the following sections, I define the particular way in which Nietzsche's madness can be shown to "speak" critically to theoretical knowledge and the history of philosophy more broadly.

In Sect. 2.3.1, "Knowledge is for Cutting", I argue that Foucault's course "The Will to Know" is an essential pre-requisite for understanding his subsequent article "Nietzsche, Genealogy, and History" and that the analysis of "de-implication" allows us to grasp genealogical critique as enacting the gesture of cutting. In Sect. 2.3.2, "The Riddle of Hysteria", I provide an elaboration and justification for bringing to bear the function of the Hysteric's riddle on Foucault's genealogy. I draw a direct connection between Foucault's passion for knowledge-*savoir* and the "castrating game" at play in the Hysteric's discourse which targets the discourse of mastery. Moreover, I present Lacan's formalization of the Hysteric's discourse as disclosing the structure of speech through which madness "speaks".

2.3.1 Knowledge Is Made for Cutting

Published in homage to Jean Hippolyte, his predecessor at the Collège, "Nietzsche, Genealogy and History" (1971) was the outcome of a series of lectures on Nietzsche that Foucault delivered in France and the United States between 1969 and 1971. In the article, Foucault states that archaeology is the method in which a genealogical purpose can be realized; it provides the necessary tools for effecting a fundamental reversal in the ingrained habits of our intellectual existence. An archaeological methodology implies a particular epistemological predisposition (e.g., violence) while genealogy connotes an ethical commitment through which Foucault demonstrates that discourse is inevitably political, the constitution of knowledge is inseparable from the exercise of power. Opposed to traditional history, Foucault defines genealogy as "effective history" in which the aim of analysis is not defined by the search for origins or *Ursprung*, but for the *Herkunft* (provenance) and the *Entstehung* (emergence).[20]

The distinction between history, on one hand, and genealogy, on the other, is significant if we consider the problem Foucault raises with respect to Aristotle in the *Lectures on The Will to Know*. One reason why the Aristotelian analysis of knowledge is important, according to Foucault, is that it set "the historical mode of existence for philosophy for centuries, and no doubt up to the present" (*LWTK* 37). Foucault argues that the history of philosophy is "always organized in terms of an interplay between the individual œuvre and a historical destination of the truth" (37). Consequently, at least two principles are assured for the history of philosophy in this regard. The first, Foucault argues, is "the inaccessibility of philosophy from the outside" since its discourse brings with itself "an ineradicable relation to truth" in which no other practice that is not philosophical can have any effect upon it (38). The second, Foucault claims, is "that of the return" by which he means that every new philosophy must think the unthought of a different philosophy which defines their singular relation to truth (37). As a result, the history of philosophy can only conceive of individual philosophies as existing in "a reciprocal relation of repetition and commentary" which preclude exteriority (37).

In his 1971 article, Foucault recalls that one can do "the genealogy of history" (*NGH* 157). This would be the "genealogy of historical sentiment" as "the genealogy of the historian's profession" which Daniel Defert describes as "the absence of œuvre" and "writing so as to no longer have a face", respectively (*LWTK* 274). By dealing with events in their unique characteristics and acute manifestations, the genealogist uproots "traditional foundations" in history and "disrupts its [ideal] continuity" as a teleological movement or a natural process" (*NGH* 154). In the same article, Foucault hints that we cannot adequately grasp genealogy without appreciating the critical imperative that drives it which he summarizes in the following way: "knowledge is not made for understanding; it

[20] Chapters 2 and 3 develop a reflection on genealogy as an analysis of "provenance" and "emergence" respectively.

is made for cutting" (154). This slogan-like statement differentiates the historian's relationship to knowledge from that of the genealogist and recalls the two paths for knowing made available by "The Will to Know".

Whereas Aristotle, in Foucault's reading, defined a certain interiority of philosophical discourse, Nietzsche situated the analysis of the *will to know* in a transgressive outside; the point at which philosophical subjectivity breaks down. Contrary to Aristotle's model which ensures the unity and identity of the subject in desire and knowledge, genealogy introduces discord or discontinuity into our very being. In the *Lectures on the Will to Know*, this is expressed in terms of "malice" turned towards the one who knows in which knowledge and desire appear in two different places, possessed by two different subjects (*LWTK* 205). Behind the act of knowledge, Foucault describes a malicious will to go "behind the surface of things" to try "to extract an essence behind the appearance" (205). Malice can also recognize that "there is still only appearance" and that "man himself, who knows is still and always an appearance", indicating the point at which the unity of the subject falls apart (205). If the passion for knowledge relentlessly "murders" all appearances, as Foucault puts it, "this work [...] is never rewarded with access to being or the essence, but gives rise to new appearances, sets them against one another and beyond one another" in an interplay of differences (206).

Foucault thus reads Nietzsche's texts as an attempt "to free the desire to know from the form and law of knowledge" (*LWTK* 25). This entails showing that knowledge is synonymous with living; one is forced into a movement where one knows to dominate, to get the upper hand and not simply in order to know. Genealogy traces the event-like character of knowledge which Foucault describes as "the reversal of a relationship of forces, the usurpation of power, [...] the entry of a masked 'other'" (*NGH* 154). From the perspective of the singularity of events, the historical development of knowledge proceeds neither from an internal necessity of what is known nor an ideal genesis of forms of knowledge. Nietzsche held that an unconscious war among its drives accounts for most of the subject's activity. It is perhaps the omission of this struggle of instincts, impulses, and desires which points to the denial and elision of a certain reality of discourse in general. Whence the "event" Foucault attributes to

Nietzsche for making desire and will emerge outside philosophical knowledge.

The Aristotelian model demonstrated the stakes of the term "co-implication" in which desire, knowledge, and truth enfold in a unified theoretical structure. In this schema, Foucault states that truth and knowledge are joined together by right; knowing is by nature, destination, and origin knowing the truth, and "truth is that which is given (or denied) to knowledge" (*LWTK* 26). Foucault presents the Nietzschean system of knowledge-*savoir* within the framework of an analysis of "de-implication". His terminological specification is useful in that it differs from the work of "explication" which would unfold the terms implicated in Aristotle's theoretical structure, but not critically. Foucault situates the properly critical act in accordance with two orthogonal directions, addressed to both: "the outside of knowing" and the "non-place of knowledge and truth" (27). "De-implication" therefore involves the introduction of exteriority using an operation that separates truth and knowledge from their original affiliation; it enacts the gesture of cutting. Through the Nietzschean path to the outside of knowledge, Foucault locates a historical analysis that would not deny or cancel the discourse of philosophy, but the position of the philosophical subject who appears *in the truth* by right.

By bringing these topics to the forefront, the *Lectures on the Will to Know* establish a potentially critical interface between madness and philosophy. Set within the broader problematic of the *will to truth* along with certain themes in philosophy that collude with its system of exclusion, Foucault presents Nietzsche as a new kind of "mad philosopher". Nietzsche's "program" of madness does not aim at the destruction of the sovereignty of reason, but the opposition of its discursive practices through a strategic detour: the outside of knowledge. There is perhaps a difference here between the "romantic" mobilization of this "outside" and its political valency in relation to the genealogical analysis of struggles and relations of dominance. Foucault's slogan-like statement "knowledge is for cutting" presents an opportunity to define the specific form that madness can take and the game it can play.

2.3.2 The Riddle of Hysteria

In this section, I provide an elaboration and justification for bringing to bear the Hysteric's riddle on Foucault's method of genealogy which I understand to be a form of "hystorical critique". To develop this perspective, I rely on Gerard Wajcman's article "The Hysteric's Discourse" (1988).[21] In this text, Wajcman tries to make sense of Lacan's proposition in Seminar XVII: *The Other Side of Psychoanalysis* (1969–1970) that hysteria is a discourse which discloses "the structure of speech in general" and "sheds light on dimensions of human discursive practices" thought to be unrelated to clinical hysteria (2003, 83). History bears witness to both aspects. In addition to clinical data, history contributes its share to describing the structure of the Hysteric's discourse. The Hysteric, argues Wajcman, is said to institute a discourse when we do not cast out her question, "a question that runs irrepressibly throughout history" (83). The notion of hysteria as a form of questioning that is profoundly historical provides a crucial link to Foucault's genealogical critique which he adapts from Nietzsche.

Drawing on the link Lacan posits between the hysteric as chimaera and the myth of the Sphinx, Wajcman presents the Hysteric's discourse as a "riddle" it posed to others. The question is the hysteric subject, <$>, whose body is marked with unexplainable symptoms. These symptoms establish the Hysteric's discourse as a question addressed to the other. The riddle of the subject supposes the other (traditionally a priest, a physician, or analyst) capable of resolving it. Beyond a clinical perspective, Wajcman states that "the history of hysteria bears witness to something fundamental in the human condition –being put under pressure to answer a question" (78). History describes the conditions under which an enigma ushers the articulation and production of knowledge. If hysteria is composed of a set of opposing and contradictory statements, then the hysteric, argues Wajcman, is what "eludes those statements, escapes this knowledge" (78). This points to the critical dimensions of the riddle.

Wajcman delineates the "castrating dimension of the hysteric's game" through reference to three key operations (88). The first involves the

[21] Wajcman's article was originally published in *Le Maitre et l'hystérique* (1982).

function of teasing knowledge (*pousse à savoir*). The hysteric begins by posing a question that demands speech: "who am I"? This entails the gesture of presenting oneself as desirable to incite the other to learn about what causes their desire. By pressing the other to use language to articulate an answer, the hysteric also pushes this other towards failure (*pousse à manque*), the second operation. With any articulated answer, the question itself disappears, as Wajcman puts it: "the subject finds itself constituted by a definite statement, 'you are…,' and the object of this statement is dropped as a lost object" (86). The hysteric is thus what knowledge must articulate but cannot, which signals the third operation (*manque à savoir*). All statements fall short of the enunciation, "in stating something it does not state the whole truth" (78). Leaving the question intact, Wajcman insists that nothing truer can be stated of hysteria than: "it is a riddle" (86).

This scenario is also illustrated in the traditional clinical context in which it has appeared.[22] Imagine a hysterical patient who presents with unexplainable symptoms that riddle her body. The hysteric's injunctive enunciation, "tell me!", enjoins the doctor to speak, to produce knowledge capable of curing her ailment. Acquiescing to her request, the physician provides a diagnosis and prescribes a treatment which the hysteric, in turn, proves to be lacking and ineffective. The next day the hysteric criticizes the doctor because her illness has not abated: the pain moves unexplainably to another part of the body. This image captures the way in which hysterical questioning poses a challenge to those who speak from positions of mastery and authority by thwarting all attempts to totalize knowledge (Fig. 2.1).

Describing the discursive relation of speaking agent to other in terms of a "castrating game" can help us to grasp the critical positioning of the Hysteric, <$>, vis-à-vis the Master, <S1>. The upper horizontal axis of the Hysteric's discourse witnesses the rise of the master. The hysteric <$> surrenders to the one empowered to answer the question s/he poses: "tell me who I am" → "I am who you say": <S1>. This corresponds to the first operation of teasing knowledge. Brandishing her suffering, the hysteric

[22] The use of the feminine pronouns she/her refer to the way hysteria was traditionally attributed to women.

The Riddle of Hysteria	The Hysteric's Discourse
Tell me who I am → I am what you say	agent <$> → <S1> other
The truth of what I am // You cannot say	truth <*a*> // <S2> product

Fig. 2.1 The riddle of hysteria depicted alongside the Hysteric's Discourse

subject incites the other's desire. At the moment the other risks a response to her advances, the hysteric withdraws only to become something other than what one thought s/he was. This provocation-turned-withdrawal illustrates the second operation of pushing the other towards failure. Having provoked the other's desire, the hysteric then disappoints it. When desire moves towards the object that causes it, the hysteric suddenly retreats and refuses to be this object, revealing the lack of knowledge in the other. By means of this third operation, the hysteric incites the other to acknowledge her as an inaccessible object of desire: "all of what I am" → "you cannot say". Putting competence into question, the hysteric demonstrates that the <S1> is always deficient.

The critical function of the riddle reveals the hysteric's ability to embody the subject and object division in a particular way. As a subject, the hysteric incites the other's desire and causes speech. As an object, by contrast, the hysteric disappoints the other's desire and resists speech. Put in slightly different terms, the subject of the utterance, "who am I", remains in the air so long as it has not found articulation by means of a statement. Once it has been stated, the object of this statement, the riddle, disappears. The left vertical axis of the Hysteric's discourse illustrates the tenuous and unnegotiable position between subject and object. According to Wajcman, the history of hysteria throws light on the structure of this discourse which consists of the hysteric's enunciation: "I am what you say" (2003, 85). History bears witness to the production of knowledge about hysteria given in the form of a statement about what the hysteric is. It also shows that no answer has settled the hysteric's question; all answers fail to master their object. In this way, history serves a vast reservoir of snapshots taken of the structure at work; it reveals the multifaceted nature of hysteria's historical guises.

Wajcman's assertion that history reveals the structure of the Hysteric's discourse as the "changing appearance of knowledge" provides an interesting overlap with Foucault's presentation of Nietzsche in his lecture course "The Will to Know" (2003, 86). In his account of Nietzsche's concept of invention (*Erfindung*), Foucault insists that knowledge is not the "operation that destroys appearance" (*LWTK* 205). Rather, it is "what constitutes the newness of appearance in the breach of appearance" (205). This claim is demonstrated by the history of hysteria. Religion, as Wajcman recalls, has shifted hysteria from "telluric demonry" to "celestial sanctity" (2003, 85). Science, in turn, classified hysteria among the organic diseases with precise and diffuse localizations, before listing it as a term or category that has now fallen into disuse. Foucault states that one consequence of these changing appearances is that "knowledge will always be a perspective; incomplete; it will never close in on itself; it will never be adequate to its object" (*LWTK* 206). Foucault's embrace of Nietzsche's perspectivism offers a preliminary means to grasp the Hysteric's role regarding knowledge and vice versa.

Similar to the question of why hysteria has remained unexplained, Foucault, citing a passage from *The Will to Power*, underscores Nietzsche's claim that knowledge can only interpret; "it does not explain" (*LWTK* 213). Knowledge introduces meaning. In many cases, it is "a new interpretation of an old interpretation which has become unintelligible" (213). Following Nietzsche, Foucault insists that every form of knowledge is the result of "an interpretive violence distorted by perspective, domination, need" (213). For Nietzsche, what prevents and constitutes knowledge is something altogether different from knowledge, that is, from the relation of subject to object. The only knowledge that is addressed to reality, argues Foucault, is the plurality of relations without subject or object. Every other form of knowledge imposes its own distortion on that reality. Far from being the truth of knowledge, the relation between subject and object is its "untruthful product" (213). Detached from truth, knowledge also fails to account for hysteria which the hysteric and her ongoing riddle make painfully obvious.

The hysteric's role regarding knowledge is ambiguous. On one hand, the hysteric solicits knowledge by presenting herself as its prized object, enticing the other to generate more. On the other hand, this solicitation pushes knowledge toward the point of failure, demonstrating that knowledge does not coincide with the truth it intends to express. It is here, I argue, that the castrating dimension of the hysteric's game intersects with the Nietzschean analysis of "de-implication" in several ways. First, the Hysteric's embodiment of the subject and object division mirrors the distance that Nietzsche put between them. Second, by maintaining a strict separation between subject and object, the Hysteric establishes a disjunction between knowledge, <S2>, and the object of this knowledge, <*a*> in the place of truth which accomplishes the aim of "de-implication". Third, due to its emphasis on transgressive desire, the castrating game of the riddle addresses itself to both the outside of knowledge and the non-place of knowledge and truth. The lower horizontal axis of the Hysteric's Discourse <*a*> // <S2> flaunts the incompatibility of truth and knowledge: "all of what I am" // "you cannot say". Like Foucault's positioning of Nietzsche contra Aristotle, the Hysteric targets a master.

This discussion allows us to envisage the critical act of "de-implication" –an act that coincides with the epistemology of "cutting" that underpins Foucault's genealogy–, through the lens of what I call "hystorical critique". It is interesting to think of Foucault's account of Nietzsche, specifically the hammer he put through the traditional theory of knowledge, as enabling the Hysteric's discourse and the mode of speech implied by it. This specific way of speaking reveals a capacity to cast the western *will to truth*, as Foucault does, in relation to a series of paradoxes in which truth and knowledge become synonymous with lies, illusions, and error. Although error is often regarded in a traditionally negative sense, as a failure to reach the truth, this is only relative to a particular conceptualization of reality. The error in one framework of knowledge may become a seminal truth in the development of a new framework. Gary Gutting describes, in this way, that Foucault's schema of knowledge as an error (or lie), is "a specific and effective counterpart to his earlier embrace of the transgressive experiences lived by the mad" (2005, 78). Differently put, Gutting states that:

> Error is itself a kind of transgression, a violation of the boundaries set by our conceptual environment. It is a localized and mundane version of the cosmic lightning flashes of madness. But what error lacks in metaphysical drama is more than compensated by its historical effectiveness. Precisely because it represents a specific deviation from particular norms, rather than an unfocused revolt against the very idea of normativity, error effects a practical change of the world we live in, not an aesthetic escape from it. In the end, Foucault subordinates the ecstasy of madness to the ironic satisfaction of (creative) error. (78)[23]

Likewise, Foucault highlights that "truth" for Nietzsche is not "something that exists and has to be found but something that *must be created*" (*LWTK* 214). Neither Nietzsche nor Foucault aims to negate the idea of truth; they strive instead to underline its event-like character by displacing a powerless truth in favor of an agonistic truth. With the categories of the "non-true truth" such as error in the forefront, Foucault defines the properly Nietzschean (or genealogical) task in terms of "thinking the history of truth without relying on truth" (217). This could also provide a formula for thinking about the function of the riddle in hystorical critique.

2.4 The Hystoricization of Truth

In the concluding section of this chapter, I want to summarize, reiterate, encapsulate and situate the key conceptual steps I have taken in the preceding section while also further situating my argument in relation to the critical context. Chapter 2 has focused primarily on Foucault's lecture course "The Will to Know" (1970–1971) and the opposition it establishes between the two theoretical models of western *will to* know, that of knowledge-*savoir* and knowledge-*connaissance*. The positioning of Nietzsche contra Aristotle was shown to present an analysis of "de-implication" that sweeps away the traditional theory in philosophy. For

[23] Gutting arrives at this conclusion through reference to Foucault's mentor, Georges Canguilhem, who, in addition to Nietzsche, provides a basis for understanding genealogical critique in the history of sciences.

this reason, I presented the lectures as a crucial reference for grasping the epistemology driving Foucault's genealogical critique which he formulates in "Nietzsche, Genealogy and History" (1971). By stressing the critical importance of Foucault's course along with the methodological shift of emphasis, I hoped to make a valuable contribution to recent scholarship in this regard whilst establishing it as a pre-requisite to his article on Nietzsche.

The chapter's emphasis on Nietzsche can be situated within wider discussions and debates on Foucault's "Nietzscheanism". Alan Sheridan, for example, highlights the foundational role of the Nietzschean will to knowledge in Foucault's work and holds that "the reactivation of Nietzsche in contemporary French thought owes much to the active role Nietzsche has played in Foucault's thinking" (2015, 118). Taking a more negative stance, J.G. Merquior tends to equate Foucault's Nietzscheanism with irrationalism and describes genealogy as "the Nietzschean reduction of forms of action or knowledge to will-to-power configurations" (1985, 143–46, 99–100). Despite his criticism, Richard Rorty holds that Foucault's thinking reflects the characterization of Nietzsche's attitude toward knowledge as an "enemy" of Hegelian historicism in that it rejects the speculative notion of historical progress (1986, 47).

Chapter 2 aligns with perspectives that locate Foucault's genealogy as a mode of historical critique in a complex relation with (post-)Kantian philosophy. For instance, Michael Mahon remarks that Foucault's concerns with the episteme are focused on the "internal conditions of our discourse, as opposed to the transcendental conditions that interested Kant" (1992, 6). The impact of Nietzsche can be observed in Foucault's thinking that the rules of formation of discourse do not refer to the transcendental structures of the mind, but those that are contingently rooted in the history of what has already been said. Although Kantian philosophy opened the space for a general critique of reason, Nietzsche removed the philosophical subject from the center of thought by orienting the task of philosophy toward a radical reflection on language, as I discussed in the section titled "Madness in the Method".

Similarly, Pamela Major-Poetzl asserts that Nietzsche specified for Foucault the limits of philosophy by assigning to it the function of "criticism, diagnosing, and demythologizing" (1983, 12). By rejecting metaphysics (as represented by Aristotle's system of knowledge-*connaissance*), genealogy remains an heir to the critique of reason inaugurated by Kant. Rather than providing a positive foundation for knowledge, however, Nietzsche links genealogical critique to a historical investigation into the falsifications of reason and the morality that underpins it. This orientation is informed by the impossibility of neutral knowledge, (as demonstrated by Nietzsche's system of knowledge-*savoir*) which enabled Foucault to think of knowledge as "a historical process before any problematic of truth" (2013, 214). In this chapter, I approached Foucault's "Nietzscheanism" in terms of the larger problematic of a hysteric(al) questioning of Kant's transcendent schema of knowledge.

Foucault's critique of "impure reason", as Thomas McCarthy notes, finds its strength in what had previously been perceived as weakness in critical theory "nominalism, descriptivism, and historicism" which serve as both a complement and "a counterweight to its emphasis on the general, the normative, and the theoretical" (1990, 463). As a mode of critique, genealogy reveals the contingency and even arbitrariness of what appears natural and necessary by relocating everything into a process of becoming. In this way, Foucault avoids metaphysical assumptions by refocusing the search for origins away from a primordial truth or original essence and toward the disparate details, events, and accidents at the historical beginning of things. Far from being teleologically oriented, the historical processes that give rise to the invention of knowledge are shown to be discontinuous, divergent, and governed by chance.

John Rajchman describes genealogy as "an attempt to lay bare [...the] consequences" of the things, values, and events that have been constituted historically, discursively, and practically (1985, 58). Likewise, Mahon explains that the genealogist constructs a counter-memory through "forgotten documents, minor statements, apparently insignificant details to recreate the forgotten historical and practical conditions of our present existence" (1992, 9). Foucault's method of critique involves opposing history to truth only insofar as truth is determined on the basis of origins, historical development, or epistemological categories of unity, continuity, and identity. Truth, Foucault insists, "has had a history within history from which we are barely emerging" (1977, 144). Genealogy traces truth's seemingly ahistorical past. In this chapter, I identified

Foucault's genealogical task of "thinking the history of truth without relying on truth" as providing a crucial link to the function of the riddle (2013, 217).

In Foucault's essay "Nietzsche, Genealogy, and History", he distinguishes the traditional model of history from effective (*wirkliche*) history. Contrary to what is traditionally thought to be immutable and unchanging, effective history accepts no constants; it "introduces discontinuity into our very being" (*NGH* 154). Derek Hook elaborates that "genealogical history is less a mirror than its opposite: a kind of opacity where we expected to find a set of historical reflections of ourselves" (2005, 22). History can be said to be effective when it estranges us from ourselves and de-familiarizes the present. This is especially evident in Foucault's theme of "dissociation" which disrupts the unity of identity of the subject by making way for a multiplicity of voices that intersect and compete in the invention of knowledge while opposing the mastery of synthesis, of "implication".[24] Disunity is also revealed in the hysteric's riddle which embodies the division between subject and object.

As a methodology of critique, Foucault's genealogy offers an array of de-familiarizing procedures that intervene in the process of knowledge production. The problem of knowledge is therefore no longer exclusively epistemic, but critical and political in nature. Foucault's inaugural course sought to determine whether the *will to truth*, given in the form of the *will to know*, exercised a system of exclusion on societies in the west. As I noted earlier, Foucault summarized his own critical imperative with the slogan: "knowledge is not made for understanding; it is made for cutting" (1977, 154). Differently put, the driving force behind genealogy is not an epistemology of truth as per the traditional configuration in philosophical theory, but an epistemology of making critique in which the critical act is one of "de-implication". The historical analysis of de-implication involves the introduction of exteriority through an act that separates knowledge and truth from their supposed original affiliation.

[24] The term "implication" was identified in Aristotle's theoretical structure to describe the way in which knowledge-desire-truth were folded together in a prior unity, removing difference and struggle from the equation.

Chapter 2 departs from the existing literature on Foucault's Nietzschean critique in that it wants to understand Foucault's positioning as a genealogist within the framework of a particular form of madness. Beyond the archaeological preoccupation with instances of discursive limitation and control, Foucault's genealogical concern targets the effective formation of discourse on "both sides of the boundary at once" (*OD* 71). Daniel Defert locates the conditions of emergence and of the transgression of discourse in what would become the "effective content" of Foucault's later teachings: "illegalities, perversions, abnormalities" (2013, 262). I raise the question of whether the "effective content" of Foucault's critical history can be shown to constitute discourse a discourse of its own, one capable of opposing systems of domination.

The interpretation of Lacan's formalization of the Discourse of the Hysteric through the paradigm of the riddle provided a starting point for my thinking around this problem. By introducing hysteria as a form of historical questioning that runs irrepressibly throughout history, Gerard Wajcman emphasizes the position of the speaking subject who appears hysterical as such. History thus plays a fundamental role in shedding light on the structure that Lacan called "Hysteric's Discourse" by bearing witness to the plasticity of hysteria's historical guises and multi-faceted nature, its changing appearance in knowledge over time. Accordingly, Wajcman highlights the hysteric's unique ability to render "unfeasible any enterprise based on the teleological organization of different kinds of knowledge" (2003, 89).

The history of the hysteria attests to the way in which the hysteric resists being apprehended as an object of knowledge, precisely because the knowledge (s)he embodies is unknowable. This factor of unknowability coincides with Foucault's embrace of Nietzsche's epistemic perspectivism which holds that knowledge is incomplete; "it will never close on itself" and "will always be separated from the thing-in-itself" (*LWTK* 206). Unlike Kant who posits that our ability to know is limited due to the form of knowledge (which is not foreign or external to itself), Foucault aligns himself with Nietzsche in claims that what prevents us from knowing is the very thing that forms "the root, dynamism, and support of knowledge; its force and not its form" (206). The force of knowledge is exterior to knowledge. In contrast to the Aristotelian system of knowledge-*connaissance*, the Nietzschean system of knowledge-*savoir* enabled Foucault to locate the transgressive force of desire on the outside of knowing. Similarly, by framing the riddle of hysteria as a "castrating game" directed at a master, one captures the transgressive dimensions of desire at play in the Discourse of the Hysteric.

The hysteric's riddle was shown to carry out the critical act of de-implication in the two orthogonal directions identified by Foucault, addressed to both the (1) outside of knowledge (e.g., desire) and (2) the non-place of knowledge and truth. The irremediable disjunction between subject <$> and object <*a*> provided a necessary condition for separating knowledge <S2> from truth <a>, revealing that the statement falls short of an enunciation; it cannot state the whole truth. The Hysteric's Discourse points to what is excluded from knowledge, namely, the hysteric subject herself. For these reasons, I considered the Discourse of the Hysteric to align with the critical imperative of the epistemology driving Foucault's genealogical critique. In other words, the function of the riddle of hysteria is not made for understanding, but for cutting down all attempts to master knowledge, challenging not so much the content but rather the position from which knowledge is pronounced "true".

If Foucault's genealogical critique makes use of the riddle of hysteria, it is perhaps only to the extent that it allows him to call into question the western *will to truth* which informs the way knowledge has been traditionally put to use in our society. By opposing history to truth, Foucault intends to reveal the historically contingent and institutionally constraining features of the true-false system of exclusion. To this end, I argued that Foucault's genealogical critique aims to hystoricize all those discourses with which truth communes: philosophy, anthropology, psychology, criminology, etc. The properly critical task consists thus in turning true discourse against itself, distorting its aims, destabilizing and unyoking it, displacing its unity with chaotic multiplicity by fabricating new histories that repeatedly weaken it. These efforts arguably begin with the hysteric's profoundly historical question: "what am I?"

The labyrinth into which Chap. 2 has ventured to situate Foucault in the Hysteric's Discourse can be read as a response to the situation of contemporary scholarship. In the field of psychoanalytic theory, attempts have been made to close the conceptual space for thinking Foucault together with Lacan. One extreme example can be observed in Joan

Copjec's (1994) *Read My Desire: Lacan Against the Historicists.* In this text, Copjec argues that historicism, (e.g., Foucault's version of it) wants "nothing to do with desire" (1994, 14). As indicated by the title, Copjec instructs historicists that, in order to develop a psychoanalytic concern for desire, they must not "read her words", that is, to register their literal meaning, but "read her desire" instead, that is, to take these words as the unique bearers of desire (189). Copjec draws on Lacan's insistence that to take desire literally is to show that desire is simultaneously that which must be articulated and that which remains somehow inarticulable.

Foucault's lecture course "The Will to Know" presents an interesting case study in this regard. On one hand, the mention of desire is unmistakable. With Aristotle, Foucault argues that both desire and the body are elided in the movement of knowledge (*LWTK* 12). In Nietzsche, desire is present at the root or underside of knowledge. On the other hand, it remains unclear what Foucault wants, if anything, to do with the role of desire. At times, Foucault appears to distance himself from the very notion of desire, seeing it not as a revolutionary force (Deleuze and Guattari 1972) but as a cornerstone for modern mechanisms of subjection. Following Copjec, I argue that it is possible to think about Foucault's words "knowledge is made for cutting" as being the unique bearers of desire in that they articulate the genealogist's specific relationship to knowledge, not unlike the critical function of the riddle in the Hysteric's Discourse. The underlying question which Chap. 2 implicitly aims to reinvigorate asks how we might re-think Foucault's relation to desire in the early to mid-1970s?

References

Andía, J. R. (2015), *Michel Foucault,* Review *of Foucault's Lectures on the Will to Know.* http://journals.openedition.org/lectures/18113 [Accessed: 20 January 2021].

Caputo, J. (2004) "On Not Knowing Who We Are: Madness, Hermeneutics, and the Night of Truth in Michel Foucault", in Bernauer, J. W., & Carrette, J. R. (eds.) *Michel Foucault and Theology: The Politics of Religious Experience.* Aldershot: Ashgate, pp. 117–139.

Copjec, J. (1994) *Read My Desire: Lacan Against the Historicists.* London: Verso.

Deleuze, G., & Guattari, F. (1972). *Anti-Oedipus: Capitalism and Schizophrenia*. Minneapolis: University of Minnesota Press.

Evangelou, A. (2017) *Philosophizing Madness from Nietzsche to Derrida*. Cham, Switzerland: Palgrave Macmillan.

Foucault, M. (1977) "Nietzsche, Genealogy, History", in Bouchard, D. F. (ed.) *Language, Counter-memory, Practice: Selected Essays and Interviews*. Ithaca, NY: Cornell University Press, pp. 139–164.

Foucault, M. (1981) "The Order of Discourse", in Young, R. (ed.) *Untying the Text: A Post-Structuralist Reader*. London: Routledge, pp. 48–78.

Foucault, M. (1986) "A Preface to Transgression", in Bouchard, F. & Simon, S. (eds.) *Language, Counter-Memory, Practice: Selected Essays and Interviews*. New York: Cornell University Press. (1977b, pp. 29–52).

Foucault, M. (2008) *Introduction to Kant's Anthropology*, Nigro, R. (ed.). Los Angeles: Semiotext(e).

Foucault, M.. (2013) *Lectures on the Will to Know: Lectures at the Collège de France 1970–1971*, D. Defert, (ed.). Translated from the French by G. Burchell. Basingstoke: Palgrave Macmillan.

Gutting, G. (2005) *Foucault: A Very Short Introduction*. Oxford: Oxford University Press.

Hook, D. (2005) "Genealogy, Discourse, 'Effective History': Foucault and the Work of Critique", *Qualitative Research in Psychology*, 2 (1), pp. 3–31. https://doi.org/10.1191/1478088705qp025oa. [Accessed: 12 February 2020].

Mader, M. (2014). *Knowledge*. In The Cambridge Foucault Lexicon. Cambridge: Cambridge University Press.

Mahon, M. (1992) *Foucault's Nietzschean Genealogy: Truth, Power, and the Subject*. Albany: State University of New York Press.

Major-Poetzl, P. (1983) *Michel Foucault's Archaeology of Western Culture: Toward a New Science of History*. Chapel Hill: University of North Carolina Press.

Mccarthy, T. (1990) "The Critique of Impure Reason: Foucault and the Frankfurt School", *Political Theory*, 18 (3), pp. 437–69. Available at: http://www.jstor.org/stable/191596. [Accessed: 12 February 2020].

Merquior, J. G. (1985) *Foucault*. London: Fontana.

Moretti, A. (2021) "Agonistic Truth: The Issue of Power Between the Will to Knowledge and Government by Truth", in Faustino, M. & Ferraro, G. (eds.) *The Late Foucault: Ethical and Political Questions*. London: Bloomsbury Academic, pp. 133–148.

Rajchman, J. (1985) *Michel Foucault: The Freedom of Philosophy*. New York: Columbia University Press.

Rorty, R. (1986) "Foucault and Epistemology", in Hoy, D. C. (ed.) *Foucault: A Critical Reader*. Oxford: Basil Blackwell, pp. 41–50.
Sheridan, A. (2015) *Michel Foucault: The Will to Truth*. Abingdon, OX: Routledge.
Wajcman, G. (2003) "The Hysteric's Discourse", in ŽiŽek, S. (ed.) *Jacques Lacan: Critical Evaluations in Cultural Theory*. Vol 1: Psychoanalytic Theory and Practice. New York: Routledge, pp. 186–198.

3

The Body's Refusal

3.1 Introduction

Foucault's genealogical method patently concerns knowledge; it concerns power, it concerns, above all, the body. The way the body has come to be reflected in Foucault's historical analyses is through a pessimistic lens, seen as something passive and lacking any agentive capacity. In his article "Nietzsche, Genealogy and History" (1972), Foucault argues that the task of the analysis of descent is to "expose a body totally imprinted by history and the process of the history's destruction of the body" (*NGH* 148). The aim of this chapter is to develop a perspective of the body that would account for the effects of social structures while also providing a critique of them in order to reflect on possibilities for resistance and transformation. To this end, I introduce Lacan's Seminar XVII: *The Other Side of Psychoanalysis* (1969–1970) in which he presents a conceptual elaboration of the structure of discourse. In line with Chap. 2, I argue that Foucault's hystorical critique articulates the structure of the Hysteric's discourse and that through this discourse we can begin to flesh out a broader understanding of the way agency and body interact in a genealogical framework.

Foucault's chronology of history, which puts into focus the transition from the "Classical" to the Modern episteme, evinces two basic modes by

J. L. Davis, *Reading Foucault Through Lacan*, The Palgrave Lacan Series,
https://doi.org/10.1007/978-3-031-69738-8_3

which discourse acts upon the body. In the Classical period, souls are separated from the body and knowledge relates to bodies through representation and direct repression. By contrast, in the modern sciences of man, there is no longer a clear hegemony of words over things. Souls are cemented back onto bodies and discourse breaks with representation to enter bodies themselves. By extension, power is no longer separated from the social field where bodies are constituted, individuated, and normalized in the interest of the reproduction of society. This shift is commensurate with the peripheral displacement of the Cartesian *cogito* by a discourse in which the material body or "thing" takes center stage, predominantly in the thought of Marx and Freud. Chapter 3 signals this modern juncture as the entry-point for bringing Foucault and Lacan into dialogue to reflect on the emphasis that both thinkers place on the materiality of the corporeal body.

Foucault argues that genealogy is a method that "attaches itself to the body", including its "nervous system, nutrition, digestion, and energies" (*NGH* 155). This type of analysis is reflected in Foucault's study of penal discourses which dictate how delinquent bodies are regulated and their interior movements made calculable. In Sect. 3.2.2 "A Genealogy of Productive Force" I discuss Foucault's engagement with the concepts of labor power and productive force in Marxian theory. I introduce Foucault's lecture course "The Punitive Society" (1972–1973) as an example of a genealogy of capitalism that traces the historical transformation of human bodies into a source of labor power. I emphasize the involvement of scientific discourses (e.g., criminology) in reproducing a power that is immanent in society, and which operates on bodies through a system of evaluation that has negative effects on the soul via the "bad conscience" which attaches itself to bodies to ensure their moral subjection.

Alongside Marx's concepts of labor power and surplus value, I introduce Lacan's notion of surplus enjoyment (*plus-de-jouir*). In Seminar XVI (1968–1969), Lacan theorizes surplus enjoyment in relation to the object of psychoanalysis (*objet a*) which he situates at the level of the discursive structure in Seminar XVII. Through a presentation of Lacan's concept of discourse as an "Apparatus of Enjoyment" (Sect 3.1) and the related understanding of the human body as an "enjoying substance", I articulate body as the surface of intersection between libidinal driving forces and external social forces. Focusing on the historical shift from the Discourse of the Master to that of the University in Sect. 3.2.1, "From *Mehrlust* to *Mehrwert*", I show how surplus enjoyment provides a conceptual means to express the libidinal dynamics at work in the social links of capitalism. I present Lacan's formalization of the University discourse as marking the historic juncture and correlation between the scientific discovery of labor power and the economic calculation of surplus value.

Section 3.3, "The New Economy of Knowledge-Enjoyment", describes the social bond of the University discourse which establishes a structural link between science and capitalism, between the accumulative regime of knowledge and the accumulation of value. With the divided subject <$> as the product of the University, I describe how powers of scientific discourses to 'invent' subjects that are 'attached' to bodies. Caught in this social mode of production and its corresponding mode of enjoyment, I highlight the position of the student-worker, <*a*>, whose knowledge is not only robbed but returned in the form of a "tyranny of the master's knowledge" which is used to intensify exploitation. I consider the cultural discontent that emerges from this situation through reference to the aftermath of May '68 in Paris. In Sect. 3.3.1 "Vincennes Enters the Circuit of Commodities", I recount an exchange between Lacan and the student revolutionaries to underscore the political failures of their actions which showcase the effects of power structures and their inability to transform them.

The post-industrial historical juncture of the University discourse raises the more general question of how relations of domination and exploitation are displaced onto things and commodities in contexts where individuals are formally free and equal. I argue that the work of Foucault and Lacan demonstrates the obsolescence of traditional models of repression for a critique of the political and libidinal economy. This is evident in Foucault's conceptual invention of "power-knowledge" which I understand to describe the modern form of what Lacan calls "knowledge-enjoyment". I assert that Foucault's analytic ability to discern the modern operation and perpetuation of power relations runs parallel to the capacity of the Hysteric's discourse to *unmask the Master's function* which concerns its relation to knowledge.

In Sect. 3.4, "The Hysteric's Labor Strike", I identify Lacan's assertion that "the hysteric refuses to give up her knowledge" as providing a preliminary basis for an articulation of the relationship between "body" and "agency" in genealogical critique. In Sect. 3.4.1 "Critique, An Apparatus of Non-Production", I explain how resistance to and transformation of the University (or scientific) discourse take place by means of the *body's refusal*, rather than its somatic compliance. Bringing Freud's case study of Dora into dialogue with feminist commentators, I discuss the paradigm of the *undisciplined body* and its refusal to serve as a means of capitalist (re)production. In Sect. 3.4.2, "An Insurrection from Below", I refer to Foucault's lecture course "Psychiatric Power" (1973–1974) to foreground his analysis of "the great maneuvers of hysteria" as a key instance of *bodies in rebellion* against the clinical apparatus of neuropathology. Furthermore, I link Foucault's discussion of "the insurrection of the hysterics" to the "insurrection of subjugated knowledges" against established social scientificity, which he identifies as the overarching aim of genealogical critique.

In the final section, "The Non-Identity Politics of Hystorical Struggle, I draw a connection between Foucault's use of genealogy and the Hysteric's discourse in that both involve calling into question the way knowledge has been put to use and made to function in society. The effective content of Foucault's genealogies, assembled over the first half of the 1970s, involves a multiplicity of bodies and resistances (e.g., illegalities, perversions, abnormalities). Their defining feature indicates a sustained refusal to embody the position of a univocal subject of science. The genealogical recovery of subjugated voices can be seen as an identification not with the "Master's 'I'" (Sect. 3.3.2), but rather with the social symptom which crystalizes the asymmetrical character of social relations under capitalist and scientific modernity. Stressing the efficacy of discontinuous, fragmented, and local critiques whose validity does not depend on established regimes of thought, I propose to grasp subjugated knowledges through the paradigm of *disunified bodies* which are free of association from the unitary body of theory and as such remain capable of opposition and struggle against the coercion of scientific discourse.

3.2 Discourse, an Apparatus of *Jouissance*

Speaking at the Paris Law Faculty at the Place du Panthéon in November 1969, Lacan announces the title of his seventeenth seminar, *La psychanalyse à l'envers*, which Russell Grigg translates as "The Other Side of Psychoanalysis" (2008, 12).[1] In the unsettled aftermath of the events of May '68, Lacan reminds his audience, many of them analysts-in-training, what his discourse is all about: "a revival of the Freudian project upside down" (12). To demonstrate this, Lacan relies on three key professions discussed by Freud in "Analysis Terminable and Interminable" (1937): *governing*, *educating*, and *analyzing*. To this list, Lacan adds a fourth term, one that addresses itself to the socio-political dynamics of the time: *protesting*. Lacan's schemata of the Discourses of the Master, the University, the Analyst, and the Hysteric provide a means, respectively, by which to apprehend these four social phenomena.

Over the course of that year (1969–1970), Lacan presents his theory of the four discourses in an attempt to analyze the crucial factors through which language exercises a formative and transformative role in human affairs. In reference to Ferdinand de Saussure's structural linguistics, Lacan insists on the distinction between speech (*parole*) and language (*langue*) to introduce his concept of discourse. Speech refers to the utterance or statement which attempts to fix meaning. Language, on the other hand, designates the general symbolic order, its system of signifiers which stand in particular relations with a central signifier, and which exist before and without the individual speaker. Discourse, Lacan states, is "a necessary structure that goes well beyond speech" (*SXVII* 12). His target is to show how "discourse can subsist without words" in certain fundamental relations that are formed and maintained through the instrument of language which is greater and more far-reaching than actual utterances (13).

That the deployment of speech "has been confused with what discourse is" contributes, in Lacan's view, to why language has been so poorly misunderstood (167). Speech is occasional; its utterances can partake in

[1] In addition to "the other side", Grigg notes that *envers* "carries the meaning of 'back', 'verso', 'lining', 'underside', 'flipside', 'underneath', and 'bad side'—connotations of the unseen even the obscene which the English translation only barely suggests", p. 9.

the imperatives that derive from discourse which are "inscribed in what functions as this reality, [the] reality of a discourse that is already in the world" (14). Before any act of speech, discourse distributes relations between speakers. By stabilizing a number of relationships among speaking beings, language provides the condition of possibility for discourse. Language is not something we can circumscribe since we are already enmeshed in it on account of our prenatal induction into a particular speech community. Lacan stresses the political undertones of this enmeshment: "I do not mean that we use it, [it] is language that uses us" (66). The presentation of discourse as a structure within which speaking beings are caught enables Lacan to articulate that "what dominates society is the practice of language" (207).

Since it involves minimally two speakers, discourse designates a social link in which the speaking being always already occupies a specific position vis-à-vis the other. Lacan bases his formalization of social links on the dyadic relationships of master/slave, teacher/pupil, analyst/analysand, and hysteric/master. The social functions of *governing*, *educating*, *analyzing*, and *protesting* from which Lacan's theory of the four discourses derives, can be understood to articulate different systems of knowledge that position speaking beings in certain ways and at certain points within those systems. The three terms (signifier, subject, object) that occupy the four places of Lacan's discursive "quadripode" illustrate how the subject-object relation is structured by language as it exists in the social convention of speakers.[2] By distinguishing the subject as a speaking being and not merely as an individual, Lacan situates his concept of discourse at the point where human beings are subjected through language.

Dominiek Hoens asserts that discourse is "another way of answering questions about the advent of the subject, the signifier, and intersubjectivity" which Lacan spells out through the use of quasi-mathematical formulae known as "mathemes" (2006, 94).[3] The intervention of the master

[2] The notion of a quadripode allows us to think of the discursive structure as having four "feet" which remain fixed while the terms that occupy the four position rotate from one discourse to the next.

[3] The matheme is Lacan's neologism for a unit of formalisation. "Mathème" derives from the word mathematics, presumably by analogy with the term "mytheme", a term coined by Claude Lévi-Strauss to denote the basic constituents of mythological systems.

signifier, formalized as <S1>, is understood as the subject's condition of possibility. According to Lacan, the <S1> is what "represents the subject for another signifier", making it possible for human beings to access the symbolic order qua language (*SXVII* 29).[4] The <S1, S2> articulation leaves a remainder, <*a*>, which Lacan qualifies as *objet a* or, that part of the subject's being which is simultaneously left out and produced by the chain of signifiers. Colin Wright explains that speaking introduces "an excess or left-over because the speaker has a real body of drives which cannot be symbolized in speech" (2016, 133). One consequence of the assumption of speech is that language produces a subject in deficit in relation to what is being said. The bar that divides the subject <$> indicates the division of the speaking being in language.

By formalizing the basic components of speech and its effects, Lacan intends to account for what is at stake when one claims the right to speak and identifies four places that come into play with every speech act. The fixed positions of Lacan's discursive matrix hold the places of (1) agent, (2) other, (3) production/loss and (4) truth. The dominant factor or agency of every discourse sits in the top-left position and indicates that which is most obvious in it. The receiver occupies the top right position whose factor is called into action by the agent of the discourse. This activation is required to receive and understand the discursive message. The bottom right position indicates the effect of those actions as a result from the other having been interpellated by the agent's dominant factor. The place of truth in the bottom left position stands for the condition of possibility that gives rise to the dominant factor but remains repressed by it. "Truth" carries the psychoanalytic insight that speech often conveys a meaning unknown to us; what we consciously intend to say is not always the truth of what we said (Bracher 1993).

Lacan's conceptualization of discourse represents a subversion of the humanist notion of speaking beings actively employing speech and points instead to failures in the imagined circularity of human communication (Peters and Appel 1996; Wright 2016). Each discourse organizes the four

---

[4] The signifier is defined by its difference from and opposition to every other signifier. The signifier can only function differentially; if it stands alone, the signifier signifies nothing. This helps to explain why Lacan posits the subject in relation to the chain of signifiers <S1, S2>.

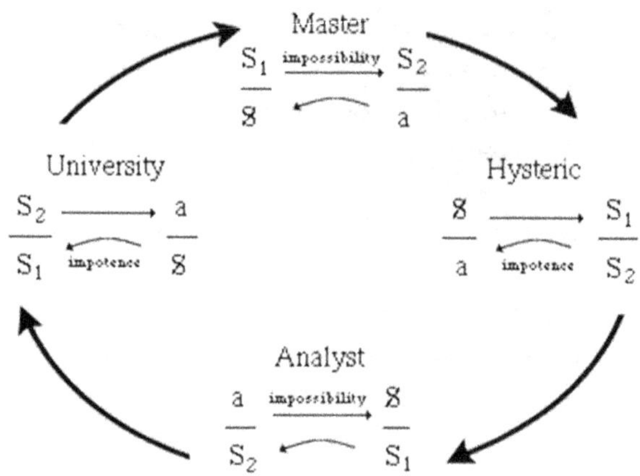

Fig. 3.1 The Four Discourses and their circular permutation

terms <S1, S2, $, *a*> in a strict circular sequence which, as Justin Clemens and Russell Grigg remark, "allows [for] rotation but no communication", meaning that changing their order relative to one another is structurally proscribed (2006, 4). Through an operation that Lacan calls "circular permutation", one discourse will be deduced from and transformed into another whenever the four terms undergo a quarter-turn (*SXVII* 39). Illustrated in the diagram below is the permutational logic of the quarter-turn represented by the discourses in a clockwise rotation Fig. 3.1.

For historical reasons and to highlight the alienating function of the signifier to which all speaking beings are subject, the four discourses begin with the Master's discourse, headed by <S1>.[5] One quarter-turn leads to the Hysteric's discourse whose simultaneous demand for and rejection of any perceived master exemplifies the primacy of subjective division, <$>. The Discourse of the Analyst emerged in the wake of Freudian psychoanalysis when it became possible to discern the structure of the Hysteric's discourse by bringing the repressed content <*a*> into the dominant position. A further rotational turn leads to the University discourse; a modern social link in which scientific knowledge <S2> is increasingly applied to the management of public life (Table 3.1).

[5] See subsection 3.2.1 "From *Mehrlust* to *Mehrwert*" for an overview of these historical reasons.

Table 3.1 A table of concepts designated by Lacan's mathemes

	Concept designated
S1	Master signifier
S2	Knowledge (*savoir*), or "knowing that–"
a	Both *objet a*, and surplus-*jouissance*
$	Divided subject

Another way of understanding the concept of discourse is to consider the originality of Seminar XVII (1969–1970) which posits an original link between the signifier and what Lacan calls "*jouissance*". The beginner is bound to encounter difficulties with the term partly because Lacan does not provide a straightforward definition, offering instead vague but often titillating indications for the reader.[6] *Jouissance*, he tells us, "begins with a tickle and ends in a blaze of petrol" (*SXVII* 72). The less than adequate English translation, "enjoyment", only adds to the ambiguity as it tends to evoke ideas about pleasure.[7] For Lacan the opposite is true: enjoyment is what "succumbs to displeasure" (77). Lacan reads the displeasure in question in relation to Freud's essay *Beyond the Pleasure Principle* (1920) in which Freud concluded that there is something beyond the rule and principle of pleasure that works against it and serves as the cause of a paradoxical repetition or compulsion since what gets repeated is not exactly pleasurable.

One implication of Freud's drive theory, as Paul Verhaeghe notes, is that "death is the final form of pleasure" (2006, 30). Continuing along the same line of reasoning, Lacan's concept of discourse accounts for the fact that "what necessitates repetition is *jouissance*" (*SXVII* 45). What interests Lacan *qua* repetition and which is "registered with the dialectic of enjoyment is, properly speaking, what goes against life": the death drive (45). Lacan refers the satisfaction proper of enjoyment to the death drive: "it is because there is the search for enjoyment as repetition that the drive is produced" (45). With its emphasis on discourse, Seminar XVII establishes both an immediate and primordial relationship between the signifier <S1> and enjoyment insofar as it is the repetition of the former

[6] For an introductory overview of the term, see Nestor Braunstein's (2003) "Desire and Jouissance in the Teachings of Lacan" in *The Cambridge Companion to Lacan*, pp. 102–115.

[7] I employ the terms *jouissance* and enjoyment interchangeably.

that constitutes a means by which speaking beings gain access to the latter (*jouissance*) (Zupančič 2006; Verhaeghe 2006).

Jacques-Alain Miller (2000) observes that, prior to *The Other Side of Psychoanalysis*, Lacan based his conceptual formulations on an antinomy between the signifier and *jouissance*, conceiving it either as a basic opposition of terms (as in the 1959–1960 seminar *The Ethics of Psychoanalysis*) or as two heterogeneous elements related by a structural analogy (as in the 1963–1964 seminar *The Four Fundamentals of Psychoanalysis*).[8] Seminar XVII is inaugural in that Lacan introduces a specific elaboration of the road to enjoyment that concerns both the formation of the subject and the subject's relation to *jouissance*. In particular, Lacan describes enjoyment as being of the order of an invasion that acquires markings or inscriptions on the body via the intervention of the <S1> (*SXVII* 19).[9] This understanding provides a link to Seminar XX, *Encore* (1972–1973) in which Lacan states that the "signifier is the [material] cause of *jouissance*", which makes it possible to approach the body as an "enjoying substance" (*SXX* 24). From this perspective, enjoyment stems from the fact that the body "enjoys" and can only be experienced as an enjoying substance through repetitions that center around bodily inscriptions which themselves result from the incidence of the signifier (Verhaeghe 2006).

The conceptual link for articulating the signifier together with *jouissance* is Lacan's concept of discourse itself. By virtue of the fact that "discourse is constantly touching on it" through the intervention of the signifier, Lacan situates enjoyment at the origin of its production, arousal, and renewal (*SXVII* 70). The four discourses convey Lacan's psychoanalytic insight that *jouissance* is an essential element of every discursivity. More importantly, the discursive dimension of enjoyment, as Alenka Zupančič maintains, "brings forward the political dimension of psychoanalysis" since it is here that the discourses of psychoanalysis pose questions about the positioning of the speaking subject within existing systems of knowledge that impose and enforce certain modes of enjoyment.

---

[8] Miller, "Paradigms of Jouissance" in *Lacanian Ink 17* (2000): 10–47.

[9] The "unary trait", which Lacan links to the <S1>, is the simplest form of this inscription; it not only pertains to the formation of the subject, but it also marks the relation of the subject to *jouissance* through the repetition of its unique symbolic identity. See the discussion in Sect. 3.3.2 under the heading "Becoming the Master's I".

Speaking about the critical dimensions of psychoanalysis, Lacan insists that:

> These reminders are essential to make at a time when, in talking of the other side of psychoanalysis, the question arises of the place of psychoanalysis in politics. The intrusion into politics can only be made by recognizing that the only discourse there is, and not just analytic discourse, is the discourse of *jouissance*. (*SXVII* 78)

It is significant that Lacan's theory of the four discourses, with its stress on the factor of enjoyment inherent to any discourse, is produced at a moment of significant political upheaval, and, after May'68, when the links between politics and desire become of prime theoretical importance. In the following section, I explore how discourse functions as an apparatus of *jouissance* through a consideration of the historical shift from the Master to the University.

3.2.1 From *Mehrlust* to *Mehrwert*

Even though Lacan takes inspiration for his concept of *jouissance* from Freud's essay *Beyond the Pleasure Principle* (1920), as reflected in the initial sense of *unlust* or displeasure, it remains a French invention, having no German equivalent in the Freudian literature. An exception can be observed in the way Lacan develops the term within the conceptual parameters of work, politics, and libidinal economy which he accomplishes in critical dialogue with Marxian insights. One key difference introduced in Seminar XVII (1969–1970) concerns the status of the object of psychoanalysis. Situated at the level of the discursive structure, Lacan now views the *objet a* in light of his theory of *plus-de-jouir* or surplus-*jouissance* which he introduced, the year before, in Seminar XVI, *From an Other to the other* (1968–1969). The outcome is a new neologism borrowed from German: *mehrlust*. The translation, which appears to take its suffix from Freud's *unlust*, is coined according to Marx's notion of surplus value: *mehrwert*.

In Seminar XVII, Lacan enlists discourse to situate the object of psychoanalysis topologically in the intervention of the signifier. His schemata of the four discourses can be understood to provide a structural basis for the logical relation between Marx and Freud (Tomsič 2015).[10] Bearing this relation in mind, the following discussion highlights the place of psychoanalysis in politics by examining Lacan's concept of surplus enjoyment in its capacity to articulate the libidinal dynamics under capitalism. I take as my focus the discursive mutation that shifted the structure of the social bond from the Master to the University; the discourses which Lacan situates on the other side of the psychoanalysis, opposite the Hysteric and the Analyst.

The perspective that Lacan develops between Freud and Marx takes place against a broader historical backdrop that accounts for changes in the status of knowledge. Going back to the ancient beginnings of the Master's discourse, Lacan centers his discussion on the philosophical context of Greek Antiquity. He identifies the slave, that is, the one who possesses savoir-faire pertaining to handcraft, as "knowledge from the outset" (*SXVII* 148). The slave's knowledge is linked in its immediacy to work since it is the thing that makes work possible. Lacan qualifies practical know-how as being "so akin to animal knowledge, but which, in the slave is not totally devoid of the apparatus that transforms it into one of the most articulated networks of language" (22). Stressing the slave's position as a speaking subject, Lacan emphasizes the transmissibility of knowledge. What he aimed to render politically suspect is the change in the status of knowledge that occurred when it was transmitted "from the slave's pocket to the master's" (22).

The structure of the social bond in the Master's discourse derives from this exchange which amounts to "robbing the slave of his function at the level of knowledge" (22). To the extent that it is transmissible, Lacan locates articulated knowledge on the side of the Master. He explains how the historical function of the "*episteme*" understood as epistemological or theoretical knowledge, results from borrowing "the techniques of the serf, that is to say, the craftsman" (21). Lacan describes this process as "a matter of extracting the essence of the slave's knowledge in order for it to become [the pure] knowledge of the master", and charges philosophical

[10] For an in-depth discussion of the "homology" Lacan posits between Marx (surplus value) and Freud (surplus *jouissance*), see Samo Tomsič's *The Capitalist Unconscious* (2015).

discourse for having participated in this extraction (21). To demonstrate his point, Lacan refers to Plato's dialogues where he observes that there is always someone who says:

> "Hey, look, get the slave to come over, that little fellow, can't you see, he knows." They ask him questions, master's questions, of course, and the slave naturally answers what the questions already dictate as a response [...] the aim is to make known what the slave knows but by acknowledging it only this derisory way. (22)

This scenario enables us to approach Lacan's assertion regarding the *objet a*; namely, that it follows from the fact that "knowledge is reduced to an articulation of signifiers" (50). This is reflected in the formulaic configuration of the Master's discourse in which the exchange between master and slave <S1 → S2> produces <*a*> in the place of *jouissance*.[11] The latter marks the point of coincidence of both a loss and a surplus which Lacan elaborates in relation to the notion of entropy. Through reference to the theory of thermodynamics, Lacan draws an analogy between the "signifying apparatus" of discourse as machine and *jouissance* as energy (81). Lacan expresses the simultaneity of the two with his claim that "knowledge is a means of *jouissance*" (50). He develops his point around the problem of knowledge as a signifying articulation which, when at work in the slave, "produces an entropy", that is, a loss of energy, a loss of enjoyment (50). The point of loss, which coincides with the incidence of the signifier, "is the sole regular point at which we have access to the nature of enjoyment" (51).

Paradoxically, this loss is also something which produces a surplus, <*a*>: "the lost object [by] which enjoyment is introduced into the subject's very being" (55). Mladen Dolar explains that the strange thermodynamics of enjoyment "revolves around the fact that the loss of energy becomes itself the source of another kind of energy" which keeps the machine turning (2006, 141). The emergence of the signifier <S1>, Lacan states, "is repeated with respect to S2", by the slave who in literal terms represents knowledge-at-work (19). The process of distilling the slave's

[11] The bottom right corner of the discursive quadripode is the site of production/loss.

know-how follows the mechanics by which knowledge becomes detached from work only to get bound up with the signifier. The subject "emerges from this entry into a relation" whereby the repetition of <S1> is propelled by the production of a by-product which gets produced in a process of recuperating the surplus (19). What Lacan seeks to politicize in the name of surplus enjoyment is that which the master receives from the slave's work:

> In fact, it is only through this effect of entropy, through this wasting, that *jouissance* acquires a status and shows itself. This is why I initially introduced it by the term *Mehrlust,* surplus [enjoyment]. It is precisely through being perceived in the dimension of loss—something necessitates compensation, if I can put it like this, for what is initially a negative number—that this something that has come and struck, resonated on, the walls of the bell, has created *jouissance*, [enjoyment] that is to be repeated. Only the dimension of entropy gives body to this fact, that there is surplus *jouissance* to be recovered. (50)

Alenka Zupančič maintains that "Lacan poses and presupposes a certain equivalence between work and enjoyment" which allows him to directly link the discourses to certain aspects of Marxian theory (2006, 162). The implication is that in work or labor there is something which is more or less identical to the status of enjoyment. Surplus enjoyment, the way Lacan intends to account for it, is "what actually happens at the level of surplus value", that of an "excess of work, surplus work" (*SXVII* 20).[12] Lacan presents the discursive process that constitutes the individual as a subject of value in capitalist society as being tied to the historical function of the *episteme* (e.g., theoretical knowledge) which amounts to a theft of knowledge. Knowledge, in other words, "is only tool for exploitation" (83). Lacan considers the situation of the wealthy who buy but do not actually pay. This is because, as Lacan argues, "what they give stems from the essence of their wealth" (83). Knowledge, he claims, is the one

[12] Surplus-value is defined in Marx's *Capital* (1999) as the difference between the exchange value of products of labor (e.g. commodities) and the value that coincides with the effort of producing these products, (e.g., the means of production and labor power). See also: Marx's *Theories of Surplus Value* (1951).

thing they never pay for. Similarly, the master does not pay for the slave's know-how (capacity for work), it is the slave who pays in surplus enjoyment. The transformation of *Mehrlust* into *Mehrwert* occurred when:

> Something changed in the master's discourse at a certain point in history. We are not going to break our backs finding out if it was because of Luther, or Calvin, or some unknown traffic of ships around Genoa, or in the Mediterranean Sea, or anywhere else, for the important point is that on a certain day surplus *jouissance* became calculable, could be counted, totalized. This is where what is called the accumulation of capital begins. (177)[13]

The discursive mutation that gave rise to the University discourse, Lacan notes, coincided with a change that brought "knowledge out of [its] localization at the level of the slave [by] virtue of having become the pure knowledge of the master, ruled by his command" (104). The new master suddenly takes an interest in accounting, in knowledge as a means of accumulation. In the place of the old master Lacan locates an "articulation of a completely new knowledge, completely reducible formally" (80). Lacan's comments combine the epistemological and political problematic of the link between science and capital. Distinct from the "disjointed knowledge" found in the psychoanalytic clinic, Lacan claims that the discourse of science "sustains itself, in logic, by making truth a play of values" (91). It is this purely logical knowledge which the University discourse puts into circulation. The social bond it institutes is more directly economic; the knowledge it accumulates is rooted in the imperatives of capital.

The University discourse marks the historic juncture and correlation between the scientific discovery of labor power and the economic calculation of surplus value. The emergence of capitalist social links requires that the product of the slave's work, <*a*>, be counted and totalized, that is, transformed into surplus value. It equally depends on a free worker selling their labor power on the market. In place of the slave, Lacan introduces the university student who freely positions him or herself within the new economy of knowledge in the place of a "more or less tolerable exploitation" (178). Lacan refers to this interpellated other as "*a-studé*", an attempt to

[13] Lacan is perhaps referring here to Fernand Braudel of the Annales school, and his work on the Mediterranean in the Age of Phillip II, which was current at the time.

work the *objet a* into the term *study* to convey something of the place the student occupies in the human sciences. Contrasting the nature of the student's work with that of the slave, Lacan observes that the *a-studé* are called upon "to constitute the subject of science with their own skin" (106).

If the individual's worth in capitalist society is defined by his or her market value, Lacan emphasizes that in addition to labor, the individual is selling out their know-how which inhered in their work all along. Juliet MacCannell explains that expropriation occurs "in the conversion of the producer's unknown knowledge into a formal value to be recuperated by and accumulated in the system itself" (2006, 201). Lacan intends to demonstrate that the University discourse reduces the student-worker to being nothing but a value, claiming that: "in the process, what you lose is your knowledge, which gave you your status" (*SXVII* 80). The world of accounting and formalizing surplus enjoyment has the consequence of devaluing the one who produces knowledge, just as the social bond in the master's discourse revealed that the knowledge spoliated from the slave had the effect of reducing the slave even more to the status of slave. Speaking to his own contribution to Marxian theory, Lacan states that:

> Marx denounces this process as spoliation. It's just that he does it without realizing that its secret lies in knowledge itself, just as the secret of the worker himself is to be reduced to being no longer anything but a value. (80)

Lacan's presentation of the social bond in the University discourse shows that "surplus *jouissance* is no longer surplus *jouissance* but is inscribed simply as a value to be [...] deducted from the totality of whatever it is that is accumulating" (*SXVII* 80–81). Knowledge <S2> accumulates by means of what is working in the place of the student, <*a*>. Given this new configuration, Lacan states that "surplus value combines with capital" (178). With <S1> in the position of truth, the University discourse is shown to represent a radicalization of the traditional master. As a result, Lacan states that "the master signifier only appears even more unassailable" (178). This is because the master now stands for value and scientific progress, making it even more difficult to stop the discursive machine from turning due to the seemingly innocent and neutral command of science "to keep on knowing more!" (105).

3.2.2 A Genealogy of Productive Force

How are we to think Lacan's account of the four discourses, with its proposed genealogy of enjoyment, in relation to Foucault's work on discourse and power? In this section, I consider the historical shift from the Master's discourse to that of the University through a different lens, one that allows us to grasp the role of the body and enjoyment as a "productive force". I highlight the way Foucault's genealogies engage with Marxian concepts through emphasis on both the materiality of human bodies and the productive aspects of power.

One example can be observed in Foucault's lecture course on "The Punitive Society" (1972–1973) in which he presents a genealogy of the prison which can also be seen as a genealogy of capitalism. In this course, Foucault formulates the conceptual couplet "*surveil*-punishment" in which he identifies a modern political strategy for imposing "a power relationship indispensable for fixing individuals to the production apparatus, for the formation of productive forces, [which] characterizes the society that may be called disciplinary" (*PS* 196). By linking the body in its biological functioning to institutional apparatuses of force, Foucault stresses the manifold ways in which the body is divided and manipulated in modern societies.

In contrast to the previous year's course lecture, "Penal Theories and Institutions" (1971–1972), which centered on the repressive aspects of embryonic State forms, Bernard Harcourt claims that Foucault "orients himself toward the productive aspects of the penal" (*PS* 280). No longer as interested in the negative functions of exclusion and repression, Foucault studies the positive effects of penal systems on the exercise and maintenance of power in capitalist society. Foucault thus brings the problem of penalty into focus within a wider analysis of political economy and the history of capitalism. In particular, Foucault develops a perspective regarding the transformation of individual labor power into a social productive force which he takes to be "the penal system's condition for being able to function in our society" (*PS* 51).

Foucault focuses on a crucial change that occurred in the historical transformation from feudal to industrial society. The main problem of feudal society, he claims, was that of "localizing individuals" by binding them to an estate for the purpose of exercising one's sovereignty and extracting rent (*PS*, 211). In industrial society the problem ceases to be "territorial" and becomes one of seizing individuals "in a temporal mesh that ensures that their life is effectively subjected to the time of production and profit" (211). The passage from "localization" to "temporal sequestration" required a range of institutional support from schools, factories, prisons, and hospitals. The control of time is the first and primary function of institutions of sequestration which organize and manage the individual's daily life and body. According to Foucault, time itself must be put on the market transformed into "working time", into the "object of wages", the wage exchange (218). The time and life of man are not, however, labor by nature; they include pleasure, desire, leisure, and revelry "—all this explosive energy must be transformed into a continuous labor power continually offered on the market" (232).

The paradigm of "temporal sequestration" demonstrates how the capitalist mode of production was organized into a new system of power during the eighteenth and nineteenth centuries. To understand what motivates people to become bearers of their own labor power, Foucault identifies "a system of power like sequestration [which] goes beyond the mode of production" and is, instead, constitutive of it (*PS* 232). The implication is that power relations do not refer to principles and foundations, economic or otherwise, but to the very action of power's constitutive mechanisms. Likewise, they cannot be described as "something located in State apparatuses" which provide them structural support (273). In implicit dialogue with Louis Althusser, Foucault resists conceiving of power as a possessable instrument or ideological apparatus; rather, power relations must be thought of as a constitutive factor, constitutive of the capitalist mode of production in that they convert the time of life into a form of labor power:

> [T]he problem of industrial society is to see to it that the individual's time, which is purchased with wages, can be integrated into the production apparatus in the form of labor power. It is necessary to ensure that what the employer buys is not empty time, but indeed labor power. In other words, it is a matter of constituting the individual's time of life into labor power. Which leads to this conclusion: if it is true that the economic structure,

> characterized by the accumulation of capital, has the property of transforming individuals' labor power into productive force, the aim of the structure of power which takes the form of sequestration is, prior to that stage, to transform the time of life into labor power. (232)

With this, Foucault concludes that "man is linked to labor at the level of his life and body" by means of a power relationship (219). Focusing on the organization of the penal system at the start of the nineteenth century, Foucault observes that "the prison-form of penalty corresponds to the wage-form of labor" (261). With prison as the general form of punishment, the body no longer has to be marked by torture but, rather, "trained and retrained; its time has to be measured and fully utilized; its forces have to be continually applied to labor" (261). This constitutes an important chapter in history of capitalism since at stake is "the transformation of the body into labor power" (218). Foucault links the problematization of the body in the history of penality to changes in the "physics of power" that occurred alongside the development of State structures. These included a "new optics" (panopticism), a "new mechanics" (disciplinary techniques) and a "new physiology" (corrective and punitive interventions) (262).

The diversity of interpellative practices control and shape the development of bodily capacities through institutional techniques of monitoring, supervising, measuring, punishing, and classifying. These techniques also depend on the formation of a certain self-relation in which workers are responsible for maintaining their labor power and allowing it to be employed and conducted in compliance with the demands of capitalist production. In *Discipline and Punish*, Foucault reads these techniques on par with the means of production themselves insofar as both are fundamental to capitalist production and the exploitation of surplus value, he states:

> [T]he two processes—the accumulation of men and the accumulation of capital—cannot be separated [...] the technological mutations of the apparatuses of production, the division of labour, and the elaboration of disciplinary processes sustained a set of very close relations. (*DP* 221)

In the same text, Foucault also explains that the "accumulation of men" coincides with the production of docile bodies:

> Discipline increases (*majore*) the forces of the body (in economic terms of utility) and diminishes these same forces (in political terms of obedience). In short, it dissociates power from the body; on the one hand, it turns it into an "aptitude", a "capacity", which it seeks to increase (*majorer*); on the other hand, it reverses the course of the energy, the power that might result from it, and turns it into a relation of strict subjection. (*DP* 138)

While the production of docile bodies remains an integral measure for converting individual labor power into a social productive force, it does not fully explain how the couplet *surveil*-punish functions as a means of ethical coercion. For this to occur, Foucault argues in the 1972–1973 lecture course that the bourgeoisie had to insert something other than "a negative law" to control working-class illegalisms: "the worker himself had to be moralized" (*PS* 147). Foucault's genealogy demonstrates that moralization is inscribed in the economic process itself. The problem posed to the penal system necessitated a solution to the question of how to free "the conditions of use of labor power" from every "hindrance and the materiality of the apparatuses of production" (175). Foucault understands the management and control of illegalisms as a way of protecting the interests and material property of the bourgeoisie.

In summary, Bernard Harcourt explains in the "Course Context" that the transformation of illegalisms into illegalities was facilitated by the value judgements of the bourgeoisie who succeeded in converting marginal behaviors into "morally blameworthy acts" and "expressions of moral fault" (*PS* 290). The practice of surveillance and control, Foucault argues, formed "the junction of the moral and the penal" in that it "established continuity between moral control and repression on one hand and the penal sanction on the other" (*PS* 107). Violations of the penal code were managed through a requalification of the working-class delinquent as someone who is in perpetual need of penitential correction who must be properly oriented into the system of capitalist production.

Following Nietzsche, Foucault shows that a genealogy of morality is indispensable to political economy and the history of capitalism. What interested him was the ensemble of political and economic processes that tied the image of the criminal to the social status of an enemy. The latter established an (im)moral basis through which to transform time and life into a productive force while fashioning a disciplinary and punitive society. The constitution of the social enemy, Foucault states, depends on "an instrument by which the class in power transfers to society [...] the function of rejecting the criminal" (36). The instrument's condition of possibility is the insertion of an institutional discourse claiming scientific status within the penal system (e.g., sociology, criminology). Foucault points here to a type of knowledge that arose "at a precise point of the relationship of worker body and force of production": examination (196). The implication is that measuring and classifying individuals in terms of their capacity for productivity depends on the normalization of capitalist social relations more broadly.

3.3 The New Economy of Knowledge-Enjoyment

In the previous section, "Discourse, an Apparatus of Enjoyment", I outlined the obsolescence of traditional models of repression for a critique of the political and libidinal economy. The present section, "The New Economy of Knowledge-Enjoyment" focuses mainly on Lacan's formalization of the University discourse which is shown to condition the social process with scientific progress. By foregrounding the productive aspects of repression with the formula "knowledge-enjoyment", I intend to throw a bridge between Foucault and Lacan. For Foucault, "power-knowledge" designates the political nexus between science, the accumulative regime of knowledge, and capitalism, the accumulative regime of value. The emergence of the University discourse in this post-industrial historical juncture raises the more general question of how relations of domination and exploitation are displaced onto things and commodities in contexts where individuals are formally free and equal.

In Sect. 3.3.1, "Vincennes Enters the Circuit of Commodities", I consider the cultural discontent that emerged in the aftermath of May'68 which provided the context in which Lacan theorized the four discourses.

I recount an exchange between Lacan and the student revolutionaries to underscore the political failures of their actions. Lacan argues that rather than subverting the master's authority, the student revolts resulted in a simple redistribution of tasks and places within the capitalist system. The establishment of the experimental Vincennes university and the adoption of a new credit-point system, founded in direct response to May '68, offered proof that the students themselves had entered the circuit of commodities. I discuss Lacan's claim that the student revolutionaries played the role of the "*lumpenproletariat*", in order to describe the function of surplus labor in a system where knowledge is progressively commodified. In Sect. 3.3.2, "Becoming the Master's I", I explain how the University discourse fosters the social implementation of knowledge corresponds to the production of capitalist subjectivity.

3.3.1 Vincennes Enters the Circuit of Commodities

On 3 December 1969, Lacan delivers the first of four impromptu sessions titled "Analyticon" at the newly established *Centre Universitaire Expérimental de Vincennes*. The latter was founded in direct response to the events of May 1968 which saw the restructuring and overhauling of an old conservative system that had previously structured Parisian universities. Following the establishment of Vincennes Lacan, who formerly held lectures at the École Normale Supérieure (ENS) in the rue d'Ulm, was obliged to relocate to the Faculté de Droit where he delivered his Seminar XVII. At the end of the decade, the social order was no longer on the brink of collapse as it had been in the previous year, however, contestation continued to be heard. On multiple occasions, Lacan's Seminar XVII was interrupted and even cancelled, and his appearances at Vincennes proved to be occasions for student agitation and protest. The dialogue below highlights one example that demonstrates the political context of the seminar.

One student, whose intervention is recorded in the appendixes of Seminar XVII, defiantly remarks that "while this little class is purring along peacefully there are 150 comrades at Beaux-Arts who are being arrested" (*SXVII* 204).[14] For this student revolutionary, and perhaps others, the will to put oneself in peril, to risk one's life for liberation, seemed to serve a far greater purpose than attending classes "on the *objet a* like this Mandarin here in our presence who no one could care less about" (204). Targeting the perceived uselessness of Lacan's theory, the speaker calls on other students to join forces with the workers in the streets to change society and overthrow some of its most cherished institutions. These calls could not be heard without first disrupting the "smooth running of [Lacan's] magisterial lecture", which the student understands to be "a fairly good translation of the decay in the university" (204).

When Lacan theorized the consequences of May '68, he reflected on the way Charles de Gaulle's government responded to student demands. Looking specifically at the action of university reform, Lacan detected a symptom of a more general function of knowledge under capitalism and its mobilization as a means of fabricating capitalist subjectivity which he illustrated in his formalization of the University discourse. Commenting on the student's alliance with the worker's movement, Lacan argues that despite their identification with the proletariat, they are more at the level of the "lumpenproletariat" (*SXVII* 190). The latter designates a disorganized and heterogenous group which occupies the position of object. Stressing the role played by the student revolutionaries in the reproduction of capitalist social links, Lacan interjects:

> If you had a bit of patience, and if you really wanted our impromptus to continue, I would tell you have, always, the revolutionary aspiration has only a single possible outcome—of ending up as the [M]aster's discourse. (*SXVII* 207)

Several exchanges later, Lacan abruptly ends the session:

> [T]he first to collaborate with this, right here at Vincennes, are you, for you fulfil the role of helots of this regime. You don't know what that means either? The regime is putting you on display. It says: "Look at them enjoying!" Good-bye for today. Bye. It's over. (*SXVII* 208)

[14] The speaker is apparently referring to a group of students who held a spontaneous class on the slums and on the politics of French politician and minister Albin Chalandon.

The transformation of enjoyment into an imperative, "Enjoy!", coincides with the historical shift from the Master's discourse to that of University. The once hidden source of value <*a*> secreted in the Master's discourse is now openly declared as what produces value for the capitalist system. Given this production, Lacan stresses the continuity of labor and enjoyment in ways that intersect with the orientation of student and worker struggles in the 1960s. One early example can be observed in the slogan "*vivre sans temps mort, jouir sans entraves*" (to live without downtime, to enjoy without obstacles) which first appeared in the brochure *De la misère en milieu universitaire.*[15] Despite advising students who oppose capitalism not to waste their time in bureaucracies, the slogan is shown to align with a more radical form of capitalist exploitation by which enjoyment has become the immediate source of surplus value <*a*>.

With his formalization of the University discourse, Lacan addresses the failures of student revolts which resulted in a simple redistribution of tasks and places within the capitalist system. Rather than representing a form of subversion against the master's authority, Lacan intends to show that what the students were rebelling against (e.g., the University) had not prevented that thing from continuing incredibly well. Speaking at Vincennes—a direct product of those actions, which was born out of a conciliation made by the French state to quell student protests–, Lacan underlines the function of surplus enjoyment that pertains to the *objet a.* The objectification of students in the University discourse, reflected in the discursive relation of agent to other <S2→ *a*>, conveys the notion of their embodiment as both surplus labor and surplus enjoyment.

Lacan's comments target those students who were directly implicated in the founding of an experimental institution and who were being counted among the regime's first collaborators. Part of the unconventional character of the university at Vincennes stemmed from its interdisciplinary programs as well as the establishment of the first ever Department of Psychoanalysis in France. The adoption of the Anglo-American valorization of knowledge at Vincennes, however, introduced a novelty in continental Europe. In particular, the installation of the credit-point system

[15] This slogan first appeared in the Situationist pamphlet distributed in November 1966 to the students of Strasbourg.

reflected a significant historical change that situated the University discourse on par with the capitalist commodification of knowledge. Speaking at Vincennes, Lacan offers proof that the students themselves had entered the circuit of commodities:

> You are the product of the university, and you prove that you are the surplus value, even if only in this respect—which you not only consent to, but which you also applaud—and I see no reason to object—which is that you leave here, yourselves equivalent to more or fewer credit points. You come here to gain credit points for yourselves. You leave here stamped, "credit points" [*unités de valeurs*]. (*SXVII* 201)

The post-industrial historical juncture of the University discourse raises the more general question of how relations of domination and exploitation are displaced onto things and commodities in a context where individuals are formally free and equal. Under capitalist social links, the accumulation of capital depends on gaining "surplus value" which, in Marx's conceptualization, is only possible by selling fetishized commodities for a price that is higher than the value attributed to the labor that produced them.[16] In the University discourse, knowledge <S2> appears as laborer, but the actual labor is accomplished by "surplus value". To put it in slightly differently terms, knowledge <S2> accumulates by means of what is working in the place of <*a*> which, in turn, confirms the total value of this discourse.

3.3.2 Becoming the Master's "I"

The University discourse depends on the social implementation of scientific knowledge <S2> which places the other in the position of object: <*a*>. This arrangement produces discontent <$> as observed in the student protests of May '68, which further fuels the creation of knowledge <S2> as exemplified in the founding of Vincennes university. Within the new economy of knowledge, the student is interpellated as the fetishized subject of enjoyment which Lacan associates with the rabble proletariat

[16] See Marx's *Capital* (2019).

and the ancient Greek helot.[17] This identification likens the student to someone who is forced to carry out surplus labor for the capitalist system. Unlike the two historical figures, however, Samo Tomsič explains that the student "must engage in a formative process to work on themselves in order to become the subject of value and enter the market of knowledge" (2015, 195). Lacan relates the process of becoming a subject of value in capitalist social links to the progressive constitution of the position of the subject of science.

Through his theory of the four discourses, Lacan shows how repression persists in and of signifiers which concern the formation of the subject. In Seminar XVII, Lacan states that "the subject is undoubtedly represented [by the signifier] but it is also not represented, suggesting that something remains hidden at this level (*SXVII* 89). In the University discourse, the master signifier, <S1> is repressed below the bar in the place of truth. The illusion of this discourse is that it pretends to have eradicated all traces of the traditional authoritarian master. The truth, however, is that the power of the University discourse hides just below the surface, repressed (or perhaps disavowed) by the agent of knowledge <S2>. Lacan also maintains that the University discourse is the one that "shows what guarantees the discourse of science" (104).

The discourse of science, argues Lacan, is "the formalization of knowledge that renders all truth problematic" (79). The specificity of positivistic science relies on a relationship of self-identity which can be expressed as a pure tautology: A = A. Scientific truth is problematic insofar as it asserts itself as reciprocal with being and imposes an injunction of self-identity. According to Lacan, it is out of "the illusion of an 'I' that is identical to itself that the <S1> of the pure imperative is constituted" (62). Lacan places this imperative at the level of the master signifier to signal the command of science by the University discourse. The call to constitute oneself as a univocal subject of science coincides with what Lacan calls the "myth of an ideal 'I', of an 'I' that masters of the I whereby at least something is identical to itself, namely the speaker" (63). The

[17] According to the Communist Manifesto the lumpenproletariat refers to the lowest stratum of the industrial working class which act "as bribed tools of reactionary intrigue". In ancient Greece, the helot was a social class that consisted of subjugated populations occupied by spartans.

"Master's 'I', that is, the sense in which the signifier appears absolute, is precisely what the University discourse is unable to eliminate from the place in which its truth is found.

The role of knowledge <S2> in the dominant position is to order the production and continuity of this "I". As interpellated object <*a*>, the student's work entails constituting the subject of science <S>. Different from the work of the slave, the student must generate a constant movement whereby enjoyment exists and persists in the failure to produce the Master's "I", guaranteeing the effect of attraction and repulsion in the attempt to reach it. The University discourse asks students to pursue a shadow of enjoyment that does not actually exist. No longer dependent on the traditional master to exert authority, the university discourse is ruled by a pure command <S1>: "keep on knowing". One point which Lacan emphasizes is that "the discourse of science only sustains itself in logic by making truth a play of values" (91). These purely numerical truths of what is countable arise from scientific knowledge and are placed "on the horizon of a new world" (80). Fleshing out the implications, Darriba and d'Escragnolle (2017) claim that Lacan introduces "an association of the cut of capitalism where the absolutizing of the market [is] inseparable from the absolutizing of modern science itself". It is precisely in this way that Lacan describes the "new tyranny of knowledge" (*SXVII* 32).

3.4 The Hysteric's Labor Strike

In this section, I argue that Lacan's assertion in Seminar XVII (1969–1970) that "the hysteric refuses to give up her knowledge" forms a preliminary basis for understanding how "body" and "agency" interact in genealogical critique. In Sect. 3.4.1 "Critique, An Apparatus of Non-Production", I explain that resistance to and transformation of the University (or scientific) discourse take place by means of the *body's refusal*, rather than its somatic compliance. I discuss Freud's case study of Dora in dialogue with feminist commentators to develop a view of the *undisciplined body* and its refusal to serve as a means of capitalist (re)production. In Sect. 3.4.2, "An Insurrection from Below", I refer to Foucault's lecture course "Psychiatric

Power" (1973–1974) to foreground his analysis of "the great maneuvers of hysteria" as a key instance of *bodies in rebellion* against the clinical apparatus of neuropathology. Furthermore, I link Foucault's discussion of "the insurrection of the hysterics" to the "insurrection of subjugated knowledges" against established social scientificity, which Foucault identifies as the overarching aim of genealogical critique.

In my final section, "The Non-Identity Politics of Hystorical Struggle", I draw a connection between Foucault's genealogy as a method of critique and the Hysteric's discourse in that both question the way knowledge has been organized and used within society. Foucault's genealogies, compiled over the first half of the 1970s, depict a multiplicity of bodies and resistances (e.g., illegalities, perversions, and abnormalities). The effective content of Foucault's analyses is characterized by a sustained refusal to embody the position of a monolithic subject of science. In my view, the genealogical recovery of subjugated voices cannot be equated with identifying with the "Master's I" (Sect. 3.3.2) but with a social symptom that crystallizes the asymmetrical character of social relations under capitalist modernity. With reference to discontinuous, fragmented, and local critiques whose validity is not dependent on established regimes of thought, I propose to grasp "subjugated knowledges" through the lens of *disunified bodies* that are free of unitary theory, and therefore, capable of opposing and combating the truth-effects of social scientific discourse.

3.4.1 Critique, an Apparatus of Non-Production

The hysteric is an important subject for Lacan in that s/he sheds light on the ways in which knowledge, truth and power converge in scientific discourses. In this section, I explore how the Hysteric's discourse not only resists but also transforms the Master's discourse and, by extension, the power structures in capitalist society. To facilitate our discussion, I refer to Freud's experience with Dora in *Fragment of an Analysis of a Case of Hysteria* (1905) where Freud discusses the appearance of hysterical symptomatology in connection with his model of normal sexual development. I then focus my attention on Seminar XVII in which Lacan presents the Discourse of the Hysteric as challenging the historical operation by which the Master robbed the slave of knowledge. Following Lacan, I show how resistance to the theft of knowledge takes place by means of the *body's refusal* rather than its somatic compliance, as Freud held. Through the example of Dora, I argue that this refusal takes the form of an *undisciplined body* which not only resisted being disciplined into the norm of a bourgeois heterosexual female subject but also refused to serve as a means of capitalist (re)production.

Discussions of the origins of psychoanalysis often mention that Freud's invention consisted in listening to his patients which brought forth the hysteric's symptom as one that speaks, and which could be interpreted scientifically. In his experience with Dora, Freud provided the insight that the hysteric's symptom is an expression of repressed desires which appear when she emerges as a woman. The process of becoming a woman can also be viewed as functioning within the space of disciplinary power. From this perspective, Freud's interpretation of Dora exposes the ways in which scientific discourse produces the hysteric subject as a subordinated being: "woman". In their criticisms of Freud, feminist commentators emphasize the extent to which Dora was a victim of patriarchal and heteronormative power structures (Mitchell 1982; Moi 1985; Rose 1985). In Freud's discourse on hysteria, we can identify an instance of what Foucault describes as the application of new methods of power whose operation is ensured by technique and normalization.[18] This is evident in Freud's remarks on hysterical attacks:

> In general, the hysterical attack, like every form of hysteria, in women recalls to action a form of sexual activity which existed during childhood, and had at that time a pronounced masculine character. One may often observe that it is just those girls who in the years before puberty showed a boyish character and inclinations who tend to become hysterical at puberty. In a whole series of cases the hysterical neurosis is nothing but an excessive over-accentuation of the typical wave of repression through which the masculine type of sexuality is removed and the woman emerges. (1963, 123–24)

At the turn of the twentieth century Dora's father, a wealthy Austrian manufacturer, appealed to Freud to cure his eighteen-year-old daughter of

[18] See Sect. 3.2.2 "A Genealogy of Productive Force".

her hysterical symptoms. The motivation for bringing Dora to Freud was to stop her from openly protesting against and thus endangering her father's love affair with Frau K., whom Dora appeared to sexually desire. Despite Freud's then novel admission of homosexual desire in young girls, he continued to uphold the standard of normality with his model of "normal" sexual development. Among other things, Freud infantilized homosexual desire by treating it as something common to all schoolgirls, which he believed to be a "precursor of a girl's first serious passion for a man", rather than a legitimate expression of sexuality (1963, 64).[19] Furthermore, Freud argued that the "formation of hysterical symptoms draw their strength not only from repressed normal sexuality but also from unconscious perverse activities", hinting that homosexuality is one such perversion (1963, 44). In this way, Freud cast the forms of repression that all girls have to undergo as "typical", that is, in order to become disciplined into the norm of the bourgeois female and heterosexual subject.

In their conceptualization of "schizoanalysis" Deleuze and Guattari (1972) challenge the psychoanalytic notion of the Oedipal complex and see it instead as the historically specific result of capitalist privatization of the nuclear family which confines reproduction to the realm of the private sphere. Here, the family plays a specific role in curbing desires and producing self-denying subjects that are primed for capitalist social relations. Bearing this in mind, Freud's scientific discourse, particularly its use of the Oedipal myth (the "natural" sexual attraction between father and daughter), is not only unsuited for grasping Dora, but also implicated in capitalist power structures. Claudia Leeb points to the "centrality of class disciplining" in Freud's case study by insisting on Herr K's sexual aggressions towards Dora which Freud dismissed as instances of "making love" (2020, 619). Like other commentators, Leeb points to how Freud's psychoanalytic discourse can easily spin off into the Master's discourse (Verhaeghe 1999; Mahony 2001; Cottet 2012) which, in this scenario, served to cover up the truth of sexual violence against women which was rife in bourgeois households.

[19] Freud describes homosexual desire in young girls as a: "A romantic and sentimental friendship with one of her school-friends, accompanied by vows, kisses, promises of eternal correspondence, and all the sensibility of jealousy, is the common precursor of a girl's first serious passion for a man".

Lurking behind Freud's interpretation of Dora is arguably the normalization of the master's male violence against the "slave" girl. On this reading, the hysteric subject is often put in the position of victim. In Seminar XVII, Lacan develops a different line of thought and insists that "the hysteric is not a slave" of the master, insofar as s/he challenges the historical operation by which the Master robbed the slave of knowledge (*SXVII* 94).[20] On the side of the Hysteric's discourse, Lacan locates a "disjointed" and "disconnected" knowledge (*savoir*) which is foreign to the discourse of science, and which resists being integrated into its "structural laws" (91). Lacan thus describes a "perfectly articulated knowledge for which [...] no subject is responsible" and which speaks all by itself in the form of an obstacle or limit (77). It is perhaps this limit that Freud's psychoanalytic discourse encountered in attempting to apprehend Dora as an object of knowledge. Instead of bringing the analysis to term, Dora abruptly terminated the session after only three months, leaving Freud with a mere "fragment" of an analysis.

In Lacan's view, the possibility for the psychoanalytic discourse to slide into the discourse mastery is the result of the desire for knowledge, which he found to be prevalent among analysts. Speaking to a new generation of analysts, Lacan maintains that "the desire to know does not lead to knowledge, what leads to knowledge is [...] the Hysteric's discourse" (*SXVII* 23). Lacan explains that the hysteric, "in her own way, goes on a kind of a strike" by refusing to give up her knowledge (94). Furthermore, Lacan criticizes Freud's notion of "somatic compliance", a term which indicates the body's involvement in expressions of repressed desires. Taking a contrarian stance, Lacan asks: "can't we see that [...] it's more of a question of *the body's refusal*?" (94). The hysteric refuses to embody (literally, to give her body over to) the signifiers that constitute her as subject. Dora's homosexual desires along with her not showing any willingness to marry, and choosing instead to focus on her studies, endangered the reproductive role of a bourgeois female subject in capitalist societies. I claim that Dora's resistance to disciplinary power takes place in the form of an *undisciplined body*. In this sense, it is more of a question of the sexual body's refusal to serve as a means of capitalist (re)production.

[20] For an outline of this historical operation, see the discussion in Sect. 3.2.1 "From *Mehrlust* to *Mehrwert*".

3.4.2 An Insurrection from Below

In the corpus of Foucault's genealogies, bodies are acted upon in discursively constituted institutional settings where resistances are rarely constructed, and struggles are not engaged. There is at least one exception to this image of bodily passivity, this pessimistic vision of agency, which Foucault discusses in his lecture course "Psychiatric Power" (1973–1974). Contrary to the Classical period where the bodies of madmen were enclosed and separated from the light of reason, Modernity witnessed the advent of the clinic, as doctors came to know the body and its organs "in-themselves". In this section, I argue that Foucault's historical analysis of "the great maneuvers of hysteria" provides a paradigmatic example of *bodies in rebellion* against the clinical apparatus of neuropathology. Crucially, I draw a connection between Foucault's outline of how agency and body interact in "the insurrection of the hysterics" and another type of insurrection, that of "subjugated knowledges". In this way, I claim that the aim of genealogy intersects with the Hysteric's discourse through an insurrection from below.

In his lecture course "Psychiatric Power" (1973–1974) Foucault argues that disciplinary power confronts a certain limit when it comes up against "those who cannot be classified, those who escape supervision, those who cannot enter the system of distribution, in short, the residual, the unclassifiable, the inassimilable" (*PP* 53). Foucault claims that the "residue of all the disciplines, those who are inassimilable to all of a society's educational, military and police disciplines" are the mentally ill (54). Among the mentally ill are the hysterics whom Foucault sees as having a capacity to resist and transform medical power. This is evident in Foucault's discussions on relations of power between doctor and patient in Jean-Martin Charcot's clinic at the Salpetrière hospital in Paris. Beneath the pathological-anatomical body, beneath the disciplinary body of psychiatry, and the apparently captured neurological body, Foucault detects a new form, that of "the sexual body" (323). Recounting an episode from Charcot's clinical demonstrations in which the scene of sexuality takes center stage, Foucault states:

> It seems to me that [...] this sexual pantomime, is not the as yet undeciphered residue of the hysterical syndrome. My impression is that this sexual bacchanal should be taken as the counter-maneuver by which the hysterics responded to the ascription of trauma. [...] So this sexuality is not an indecipherable remainder but the hysteric's victory cry, the last maneuver by which they finally get the better of the neurologists and silence them: if you want symptoms too, something functional; if you want to make your hypnosis natural and each of your injunctions to cause the kind of symptoms you can take as natural [...] then you really will have to hear what I say and see what I do! (*PP* 322)[21]

Foucault's account of the "sexual body" offers another means by which to grasp the *body's refusal.* The introduction of sexuality in this scenario, claims Foucault, does not derive from the power of the doctors, but from the hysterics themselves, as their putting into play a point of resistance within the strategic field of existing power relations.[22] Setting aside the scientific-epistemological notion of an epidemic of hysteria, Foucault analyzes what he calls the "great maneuvers of hysteria" in terms of a "battle, confrontation, reciprocal encirclement [...] of investment and counter-investment of struggle for control between doctors and hysterics" (*PP* 308). Significantly, Foucault understands the appearance of hysterical "simulation" not as a pathological phenomenon, but as a struggle which becomes the "militant underside of psychiatric power" and in which the hysterics emerge as "the true militants of anti-psychiatry" (254). Foucault's claims are historically illustrated by the fact that during the 1880s "simulation" led to a crisis in psychiatry when the study of hysterical symptoms, specifically by Charcot and his team of all-male doctors, were falsified by the patients' simulation.

[21] In response to the medical need to find an aetiology of hysteria that will give its symptoms a pathological status, Foucault argues that the hysterics responded with the counter-manoeuvre of recounting their sexual life, with all of its possible traumatism, in order to effectuate a redistribution of force relations and a new configuration of power, p. 322.

[22] Later, in the *History of Sexuality vol. 1*, Foucault states that the effects of an initially disruptive recounting of sexual life by the hysteric will be reorganized by a scientific modality (e.g., *scientia sexualis*) of confession; the traumas of sexuality will become integrated into procedures of individualization that produce subjection. Foucault will thus single out the way the hystericization of women's bodies with respect to sex attained a historically noteworthy efficacy in the order of power, and productivity in the order of knowledge.

Simulation, for Foucault, refers to the way hysteria simulates hysteria: "the way in which the true symptom is a certain way of lying and the way in which the false symptom is a way of truly being ill" (*PP* 135). Despite their somatic involvement in simulations, I argue that Foucault's description of the "insurrection of the hysterics" as a process by which patients tried to "evade psychiatric power" through "the phenomenon of struggle", provides a paradigmatic example of *bodies in rebellion* (137). Hysterical simulation was a means of resisting the scientific attempt to fix "madness" in reality, as Foucault put it: "if you claim to possess truth once and for all in terms of an already constituted knowledge [...] I will install falsehood in myself" (136).[23] Foucault situates the hysterics at the juncture of a limit in the discourse of science which reintroduces the question of truth that psychiatry had firmly established on its side. Through his account of simulation, Foucault captures the agentive capacity of the bodies of hysterics to not only resist but also expose the truth of psychiatric classifications whose general aim was not to cure patients but to put them back to work for the capitalist system.

How are we to understand Lacan's comments about the hysteric's labor strike in the context of Foucault's genealogies? To respond to this question, I first consider the hysterics' insurrection alongside another type of insurrection, that of "subjugated knowledges". The first mention of this term comes from "Two Lectures" given in 1976 in which Foucault identifies "the insurrection of subjugated knowledges" as the overarching aim of genealogy (*PK* 84).[24] Reflecting on the instability of the social order in France over the preceding years, Foucault observes the emergence of an "increasing vulnerability to criticism of things, institutions, practices and discourses" (80). Foucault had in mind a variety of events including the student uprisings, the anti-psychiatry movement, and attacks on the legal

[23] The body's refusal in this instance reflects a refusal to embody the signifier "mad".

[24] The "Two Lectures", translated in *Power/Knowledge: Selected Interviews and Other Writings* (1980), were first published in Italian in *Microfisica del potere*, Eianaudi, 1977; they are translated into French in Foucault's *Dits et Écrits vol. II* (Gallimard, 2001), pp. 160–174 and 175–189. The "chronology" by Daniel Defert in Vol. 1 of the *Dits et Écrits* (2001) mentions that these texts were widely circulated among the Italian "autonomist" and German "alternative" groups and would inflect the political reception of Foucault's work (p. 71). The two lectures are also published in the first English-language volume of Foucault's lecture courses: *Society Must be Defended*.

and penal system—all of which are perhaps "most intimately related to our bodies and to our everyday behavior" (80).

For Foucault, the uncoordinated and even fragmentary occurrence of such polemics does not pose a problem; within anti-psychiatry, the lack of any systematic coordination or overriding system of reference proved to be less important than its potential to produce a variety of autonomous critiques (Hook 2005). On the contrary, Foucault points to the astonishing "efficacy of discontinuous, particular and local criticisms" whose validity remained independent of the approval of "established regimes of thought" (*PK* 81). According to Foucault, these critiques were only made possible through the "insurrection of subjugated knowledges" (84). Embedded in this genealogical notion are two conjoined ideas. The first concerns the use of historical contents that have been neglected and actively deprioritized by the organizing structures of orthodox systems of knowledge and theory. The second concerns a fragmented variety of non-conceptual and hierarchically inferior knowledges that have been disqualified from the sciences. These include the local, regional, and differential knowledges of the subjugated (e.g., the "psychiatrized", the patient, the perverse, the delinquent, the ill).

As a method of critique, Foucault states that genealogy opposes subjugated knowledges to a "unitary body of theory which would filter, hierarchize and order them in the name of some true knowledge and some arbitrary idea of science and its object" (*PK* 83). Foucault thus characterizes genealogy as an "anti-science" while insisting that its overall objective is to combat the centralizing power effects linked to the functioning of institutions and social scientific discourses. The combination of reactivated historical contents (via the tools of meticulous, technical expertise) alongside a set of rejected knowledges (e.g., local memories), provides vital resources for genealogical critique to disrupt the dynamic of power and knowledge. Like the great maneuvers of hysteria, what interests Foucault about these knowledges is that they remain, to an extent, inassimilable, that is, not yet integrated into the power-knowledge circuit. In contrast to projects which aim to inscribe knowledges in the hierarchal order of power associated with science, Foucault describes genealogy as an attempt to "emancipate historical knowledges from that subjection" in order to render them "capable of opposition and of struggle" (85).

Through the insurrection of subjugated knowledges, Foucault shows that it is only in contexts of exclusion and disqualification, contexts marked by conflict and the violence of marginalization, that knowledge can function as a political force.

Foucault presents genealogy as a critical and strategic approach to the project of knowledge production in modern society. The genealogical recovery of subjugated voices occurs under the auspices of tracing discursive formations of power and control. It assembles a strategically organized ensemble of historical struggles through which to interrogate the role that various forms of knowledge have in the ordering of a given social formation. Foucault's method of genealogy plays delegitimized knowledges against the power-effects of established social scientificity. In other words, genealogy, as Foucault understands it, aims primarily at the generation of critique rather than the cultivation of knowledge. The critical impetus driving Foucault's genealogy emphasizes the practical, polemical, and oppositional use of historical knowledges that are capable of contestation. Foucault's characterization of genealogy as an anti-science suggests a critical positioning vis-à-vis the University discourse. Moreover, the insurrection of subjugated knowledges reflects Lacan's claim in Seminar XVII that the Hysteric's discourse does not "testify to the fact that what is inferior is down below" (*SXVII* 94).

The inverted relation of discourse, visually represented in Lacan's formulae, is crucial for understanding the Hysteric's position of critique against the University. A further translation of *envers*, as in the title of Lacan's Seminar XVII, is "lining" (as of a jacket). From this perspective, the Hysteric can be thought of as turning the University discourse inside out.

3.4.3 The Non-Identity Politics of Hystorical Struggle

The focus of Chap. 3 has been to develop a notion of the body that would account for the effects of social structures while, at the same time, providing a critique of them. I achieved this by staging a critical encounter between the University discourse, on one hand, and the Hysteric's discourse, on the other. Through a discussion of Freud's experience with

Dora, I showed how the scientific discourse on hysteria functioned within the space of disciplinary power. This enabled me to reflect the figure of the hysteric through the paradigm of an *undisciplined body* which was shown to resist normalization and the capitalist mode of (re)production. Foucault's historical analysis of the maneuvers of hysteria in the nineteenth century brought forth the image of the sexual body which had been buried in functional coherences and formal systematizations of accumulated medical knowledge. This allowed me to explain the insurrection of the hysterics against the clinical apparatus of neuropathology through the paradigm of *bodies in rebellion*. I presented these examples as a means of grasping the *body's refusal* which I discussed under the heading, "The Hysteric's Labor Strike".

In this chapter I argued that Foucault's hystorical critique articulates the structure of the Hysteric's discourse, and that through this discourse we can begin to flesh out a broader understanding of the way "agency" and "body" interact in a genealogical framework. I formulated this argument at different points and in multiple stages while relying on Lacan's presentation of the Hysteric's discourse in Seminar XVII. One assertion Lacan makes is that the Hysteric's discourse "reveals the Master's discourse's relation to *jouissance* in the sense that in it, knowledge [S2] in is the place of *jouissance*" (*SXVII* 94). In Foucault, I maintain that this translates into the genealogical detection of apparatuses of power-knowledge which account for the productive aspects of repression in modern society. As an example, I referred to Foucault's genealogy of capitalism in "The Punitive Society" (1972–1973). In this course, Foucault traces the process by which human bodies are first converted into subjects bearing labor power and then organized collectively into a social productive force to be measured. This was explained through reference to the way discipline maximizes the forces of the body in terms of economic utility while diminishing these same forces to ensure its obedience.

Another sense in which Lacan describes the Hysteric's discourse is through the *body's refusal*, claiming that: "in following the effect of the master signifier, the hysteric is not a slave" (*SXVII* 94). I understand Lacan's comment to signal the difference between, on one hand, an interrogation of master signifiers in the form of bodily inscriptions and, on the other hand, a refusal to give body to them. Lacan also holds that unlike the slave, whose *savoir-faire* was distilled into the master's theoretical knowledge, the hysteric goes on a strike and refuses to give up her knowledge. These two points can help to clarify genealogy (1) as an analysis of descent which interrogates the body as a "surface", a set of multidirectional "forces", and as a scene or site where regimes of knowledge and power inscribe themselves, and (2) as an insurrection of subjugated knowledges against a unitary body of theory that would try to order it in the name of true knowledge or an arbitrary idea of what constitutes science and its objects.

The effective content of Foucault's genealogies, assembled over the first half the 1970s, involves a multiplicity of bodies and resistances. Their essential feature indicates a sustained refusal to embody the position of a univocal subject, of a signifier that would be its own signified. The reemergence of subjugated knowledges can be seen as an identification with a social symptom which crystallizes the asymmetrical character of social relations under capitalist and scientific modernity. Rather than becoming the "Master's 'I'", Foucault's genealogies resurface the embodiments of damaged and exploited subjectivity through illegalisms, perversions, abnormalities and the mentally ill, conveys the broader notion that knowledge is never innocent, apolitical, or decontextualized. The efficacy of discontinuous, fragmented, and local forms of criticisms can help us to think about how the insurrection of subjugated knowledges wages its rebellion via *disunified bodies* which are free of association from the unitary body of theory and as such remain capable of opposition and struggle against the coercion of social scientific discourses and the effects intrinsic to their power.

Foucault's genealogical recovery of subjugated voices is closely related to the social movements of the 1960s that called for the recognition of the dignity of Black people, women, gay men, lesbians, working-class people, and other marginalized groups. In our contemporary present, this is most associated with identity politics. Contrary to the latter, however, Foucault's historical analysis of the prisoner, the mentally ill, the abnormal, and the like acquire their combative force not by identifying with some positive feature of identity, but the obverse, a negative feature of non-identity. Hysteria, among other things, poses the insoluble question of identity, "What am I?", through its discourse. The "hystorical critique" of Foucault can be viewed as a means of questioning the way in which knowledge and truth are put to use and made to function in society. From a genealogical perspective, knowledge must become as a tactical weapon of considerable value in political struggles. Rather than being a commodity valued by the capitalist system, the hysteric's knowledge stands for that which does not fit, that which does not work.

References

Bracher, M. (1993) *Lacan, Discourse, and Social Change: A Psychoanalytic Cultural Criticism*. Ithaca: Cornell University Press.

Braunstein, N. (2003) "Desire and Jouissance in the Teachings of Lacan", in Rabate, J. M. (ed.) *The Cambridge Companion to Lacan*. Cambridge: Cambridge University Press, pp. 102–115.

Clemens, J., & Grigg, R. (Eds.) (2006). *Jacques Lacan and the Other Side of Psychoanalysis: Reflections on Seminar XVII*. Durham, NC: Duke University Press.

Cottet, S. (2012) *Freud and the Desire of the Psychoanalyst*. London: Karnac.

Darriba, V., & D'escragnolle, M. (2017) "The Presence of Capitalism in Lacan's Theory of Discourse", *Ágora: Estudos em Teoria Psicanalítica*, 20 (2), pp. 543–558. Available at: https://doi.org/10.1590/1809-44142017002012 [Accessed: 12 February 2020].

Dolar, M. (2006) Hegel as the Other Side of Psychoanalysis, in Grigg, R., & Clemens, J. (eds.) *Jacques Lacan and the Other Side of Psychoanalysis: Reflections on Seminar XVII*. Durham: Duke University Press, pp. 129–154.

Foucault, M. (1977) "Nietzsche, Genealogy, History", in Bouchard, D. F. (ed.) *Language, Counter-memory, Practice: Selected Essays and Interviews*. Ithaca, NY: Cornell University Press, pp. 139–164.

Foucault, M. (1980) *Power/Knowledge: Selected Interviews and Other Writings 1972–1977*. New York: Pantheon.

Foucault, M. (1995) *Discipline and Punish: The Birth of the Prison*. Translated from the French by A. Sheridan. New York: Vintage Books.

Foucault, M. (2008) *Psychiatric Power: Lectures at the Collège de France, 1973–1974*, Lagrange, J. (ed.). Translated from the French by G. Burchell. New York: Picador.

Foucault, M.. (2015) *The Punitive Society: Lectures at the Collège de France 1972–1973*, Harcourt, B., Ewald, F., Fontana, A., & Davidson, A. (eds.). Translated from the French by G. Burchell. Basingstoke: Palgrave Macmillan.

Freud, S. (1937) "Analysis Terminable and Interminable", in Strachey, A., & Tyson, A. (eds.) *Moses and Monotheism: An Outline of Psycho-Analysis and Other Works*. Translated from the German by J. Strachey. London: The Hogarth Press and the Institute of Psycho-Analysis, pp. 211–253.

Freud, S.(1963) "General Remarks on Hysterical Attacks (1909)", in Freud, S., & Rieff, P. (eds.) *Dora: An Analysis of a Case of Hysteria*. New York: Collier, pp. 123–124.

Grigg, R. (2008) *Lacan, Language, and Philosophy*. New York: SUNY Press.

Hoens, D. (2006) "Toward a New Perversion: Psychoanalysis", in Grigg, R., & Clemens, J. (eds.) *Jacques Lacan and the Other Side of Psychoanalysis: Reflections on Seminar XVII*. Durham: Duke University Press, pp. 88–104.

Hook, D. (2005) "Genealogy, Discourse, 'Effective History': Foucault and the Work of Critique", *Qualitative Research in Psychology*, 2 (1), pp. 3–31. https://doi.org/10.1191/1478088705qp025oa. [Accessed: 12 February 2020].

Lacan, J. (1998*) The Seminar XX, Encore: On Feminine Sexuality, the Limits of Love and Knowledge*, Miller, J. A. (ed.). Translated from the French by B. Fink. New York: W. W. Norton & Company.

Lacan, J. (2007) *The Seminar of Jacques Lacan, Book XVII: The Other Side of Psychoanalysis, 1969–1970*, Miller, J. A. (ed.). Translated from the French by R. Grigg. New York: W.W. Norton and Company.

Leeb, C. (2020) "The Hysteric Rebels: Rethinking Radical Socio-Political Transformation with Foucault and Lacan", *Theory & Event*, 23 (3), pp. 607–640.

Maccannell, J. F. (2006) "More Thoughts for the Times on War and Death: The Discourse of Capitalism in Seminar XVII", in Grigg, R., & Clemens, J. (eds.) *Jacques Lacan and the Other Side of Psychoanalysis: Reflections on Seminar XVII*. Durham: Duke University Press, pp. 195–215.

Mahony, P. J. (2001) *Psychoanalysis and Discourse*. London: Brunner-Routledge.

Marx, K. (1951). *Theories of Surplus Value: a selection from the volumes published between 1905 to 1910 as Theorien uber den Mehrwert,* Kautsky, K. (ed.). London: Lawrence & Wishart.

Marx, K. (2019) *Capital: a Critique of Political Economy*. Oxford: Benediction Classics.

Miller, J.-A. (2000) "Paradigms of Jouissance", *Lacanian Ink,* 17, pp. *10–47.*

Mitchell, J., *&* Rose, J. (eds.) (*1982) Feminine Sexuality*. Jacques Lacan and the École *Freudienne*. London: Macmillan Press Ltd
Moi, T. (1985) "Representation of Patriarchy: Sexuality and Epistemology in Freud's Dora", in Bernheimer, C., & Kahane, C. (eds.) *Dora's Case Freud–Hysteria–Feminism*. West Sussex: Columbia University Press, pp. 181–199.
Peters, M., & Appel, S. (1996) "Positioning Theory: Discourse, The Subject and the Problem of Desire", *Social Analysis*, 40, pp. 120–141. Available at: http://www.jstor.org/stable/23171700 [Accessed: 12 February 2020].
Rose, J. (1985) "Dora: Fragment of an Analysis", in Bernheimer, C., & Kahane, C. (eds.) *Dora's Case Freud–Hysteria–Feminism*. West Sussex: Columbia University Press, pp. 128–148.
Tomšič, S. (2015) *The Capitalist Unconscious: Marx and Lacan*. London: Verso.
Verhaeghe, P. (*1999*) *Does* the *Woman Exist*? From *Freud's Hysteric* to *Lacan's Feminine*. Translated from the French by *M. D. RY.* New York: Other Press.
Verhaeghe, P. (2006) "Enjoyment and Impossibility: Lacan's Revision of the Oedipus Complex", in Grigg, R., & Clemens, J. (eds.) *Jacques Lacan and the Other Side of Psychoanalysis: Reflections on Seminar XVII*. Durham: Duke University Press, pp. 29–50.
Wright, C. (2016) "Discourse and the Master's Lining: A Lacanian Critique of the Globalizing (Bio)Politics of the Diagnostic and Statistical Manual", in Tomšič, S., & Zevnik, A. (eds.), *Jacques Lacan: between Psychoanalysis and Politics*. London: Routledge.
———. (2006) "When Surplus Enjoyment Meets Surplus Value", in Grigg, R., & Clemens, J. (eds.) *Jacques Lacan and the Other Side of Psychoanalysis: Reflections on Seminar XVII*. Durham: Duke University Press, pp. 155–178.

4

Foucault's Theatre of War

4.1 Introduction

Foucault's description of genealogy relies on Nietzschean accounts of the violent beginnings of human culture. This is evident in the struggle and division inherent in the analysis of *Entstehung* or "emergence" which is based on Nietzsche's vocabulary in *The Genealogy of Morals*. In "Nietzsche, Genealogy and History" (1971) Foucault argues that the aim of emergence is to foreground the historical "entry of forces, their eruption, the leap from the wings to the center stage" (*NGH* 149–50). Due to the orientation of genealogy which traces patterns of domination to their moments of emergence, the analytical language best suited for grasping history is the thematic of constant war, the ongoing interrelation of a multiplicity of forces. In this chapter, I develop a view of Foucault's staging of war from the perspective which brings into focus the binary structure of the modern discursive field as an ongoing struggle between the psychoanalytic "forces" of hysterical desire versus perverse drive. I argue that Foucault's "theatre of war" enables us to view his genealogies as existing in a circular relation with systems of power which reveal not static states of domination but a reciprocal incitation and struggle, a permanent provocation that illustrates the agonism of history.

J. L. Davis, *Reading Foucault Through Lacan*, The Palgrave Lacan Series,
https://doi.org/10.1007/978-3-031-69738-8_4

In the early 1970s, critiques of the Oedipus complex were prevalent amongst French intellectuals including Lacan, Deleuze and Guatarri, as well as Foucault. Section 4.2., "Two Readings of Oedipus", presents Lacan's and Foucault's attempts to displace the Freudian account of the origins of human culture. In place of a universal theory, I stress the emphasis that both thinkers put on the question of contingency, the accidental, and the "alea" or chance. I introduce Foucault's historical account of the fall of Oedipus, the (Assyrian) king, and the rise of Athenian democracy, under the heading "Power-Knowledge Nexus" to underscore how each episode of emergence produces a new dispersion of rules, dominations, and contingent truths which determine the discursive space. The title "Freud's Father Complex" frames Lacan's efforts to disprove the claim that psychoanalysis transmits the reference to the (im)purity of its origins which he criticizes by emphasizing, among other things, the contingency of Freud's singular relationship to his father, as reflected in a peculiar trend in some of his clinical case studies.

Section 4.2 positions Chap. 4 in dialogue with Chap. 2 in several ways. First, it establishes recourse to Foucault's Collège course "The Will to Know" (1970–1971) through reference to his lecture "Oedipal Knowledge", which I discuss in relation to a later version of his account of the Oedipus story in "Truth and Juridical Forms" (1974). Second, it refers to Lacan's Seminar XVII: *The Other Side of Psychoanalysis* (1969–1970) where Lacan introduces his theory of the four discourses as a counter to and structural replacement of Freud's Oedipus complex. I explain how Lacan accounts for hysterical desire as a relationship that the hysteric has with a master whose truth s/he reveals to be castrated or deficient, along with Freud's father figures. Parallel to the hysteric's repeated staging of the scene of truth, I identify Foucault's analysis of emergence as an attempt to dispel the notion of historical endpoints by staging the scene of "endlessly repeated dominations" (*NGH* 150). Emphasizing the genealogist's commitment to tracing the "flows of history", I return to the themes and questions put forward in Chap. 1 concerning Foucault's relationship to desire in the early to mid-1970s.

In Sect. 4.3, "Read my Desire as a Testing Game", I turn to Foucault's lecture course "Society Must be Defended" (1975–1976) to grasp the genealogical use of history not only as a means of reporting struggle but also as a political tool and weapon in ongoing struggles. To develop this perspective, I discuss Foucault's interest in the "historico-political discourse of war" which he opposes to the dominant "philosophico-juridical discourse" of sovereignty and law in western political thought and analysis. In Sect. 4.3.1, "Recourse to Ancient Rights", I draw a parallel between the binary structure of war and the old formula of the duel in "Truth and Juridical Forms" which designates a tête-à-tête combat fought between two warriors without the intervention of any political authority to function above their heads as Law. I claim that the "testing game" offers a preliminary framework to account for expressions of hysterical desire in Foucault in that it implies both a dyadic relation with a master and a direct challenge.

By raising the notion of a "testing game" in the context of the course "Society Must be Defended", I situate it in proximity with Foucault's historical critique of sovereignty and, by extension, the position of mastery. In Sect. 4.3.2, "Truth in the Discourse of War", I connect Foucault's criticism of political sovereignty to the aspiration for "epistemic sovereignty", a term designated by the quest for the status of science in the French intellectual context. Insisting on the partial character of truth in the historico-political discourse of war, I consider the genealogical principle of sacrifice which foregoes the belief in the neutrality, objectivity, or disinterestedness of the subject of knowledge. With the term "epistemic sovereignty", I shift the discussion from the philosophico-juridical discourse to the discourse of science. Section 4.4, "The Binary Structure of the Modern Discursive Arena" is an attempt to abandon the standpoint of sovereignty in favor of the binary structure of the testing game. I show that Foucault positions his genealogies in a combative relation vis-à-vis the University discourse in which the clash of forces takes place between hysterical desire and perverse drive.

Chapter 4 marks the end of Part I: "The Hysteric's Discourse". In the final Sect. 4.5 "Staging an Exit", I consider the possibilities, for Foucault, of exiting this discourse and by extension, the problematic of war. I consider how Foucault's critique of "epistemic sovereignty" broaches the political and ethical problems involved in ridding oneself of the master's knowledge and the master's reason.

4.2 Two Readings of Oedipus

The axis of discussion in this section revolves primarily around a critique of Freud's Oedipus complex. It is divided into two parts, each outlining the attempts by Lacan and Foucault to displace the universal theory at the heart of the Freudian perspective. In the section titled "Freud's Father Complex", I bring into focus two aspects of Lacan's criticism of Freud in Seminar XVII (1969–1970). The first concerns his claim that the Oedipus complex is "Freud's dream" by which he means that it can be re-interpreted so as to allow its latent content to surface. This "latent content" pertains to Freud's singular relationship to his father in which Lacan introduces the theme of patricide. Through reference to some of Freud's clinical case studies, I highlight Lacan's argument that Freud's patricidal theme presents a defense against the fact of the father's castration which concerns his actual limitations. The second aspect, related to the first, concerns Freud's case study of Dora. Lacan develops the view that Freud's use of the Oedipus complex failed to account for the relationship between the hysteric and a master figure whose truth s/he shows to be castrated, along with Freud's father figures.

The section "Power-Knowledge Nexus" presents Foucault's account of Oedipus, the Assyrian King, in his lecture "Oedipal Knowledge" (1971) which I discuss in relation to a later version "Truth and Juridical Forms" (1974). Situated in a historical dimension, Foucault shifts the Freudian emphasis away from "Oedipus the Incestuous" or "Oedipus the Parricidal" and toward "Oedipus the Tyrant", the professional of political power who existed in the Athenian society of Sophocles' era. In this way, I explain how Foucault presents the Oedipal theme in its historical links to the problem of kingship around the dawn of Greek democracy. From this perspective, Foucault situates the Oedipus complex at the collective level in connection with power and knowledge. According to Foucault, what gets played out in the Oedipal story is a struggle between kinds of knowledge (*savoir*) and kinds of power, a struggle between power-knowledge which resulted in a new constraint of truth which Foucault sought to problematize in the west.

4.2.1 Freud's Father Complex

At the start of Seminar XVII: *The Other Side of Psychoanalysis* (1969–1971) Lacan describes his discourse as "a revival of the Freudian project upside down" (*SXVII* 12). This comment points to the critical dimensions underlying Lacan's return to Freud's original texts which is explicit in a cluster of lectures grouped under the title "Beyond the Oedipus Complex". In its merciless criticism of the Freudian perspective, this chapter has been read by some as illustrating an attempt on Lacan's part to progressively de-oedipalize his own theory (Van Haute and Geyskens 2016). Lacan's attack is twofold. First, he recasts the Oedipus complex as "Freud's dream" by which he means that Freud's theoretical construction can be reinterpreted for what it disguises and ultimately obscures so as to allow its latent content to surface (*SXVII* 135). Second, Lacan refers to Freud's case study of Dora to show how the Oedipus complex is unable to account for the relationship between the hysterical patient and the master figure. In response to these limitations, and guided by his understanding of hysteric's desire, Lacan introduces his theory of the four discourses as a structural replacement of and counter to Freud's formulation of the Oedipus complex.

Although Freud's earliest mention of the Oedipal problematic comes from his letters to Wilhelm Fleiss, a more rigorous engagement with Sophocles' tragedy, *Oedipus Rex*, can be found in *The Interpretation of Dreams* (1900). In Freud's reading, the Oedipus legend derives its meaning from the realisation of two inextricable desires: (1) the desire to sleep with the mother and (2) the desire to kill the father. Stressing the universal power of the legend, Freud developed his own hypothesis regarding the psychology of children which he advanced with an equal universal validity. To demonstrate how the Oedipus myth continues to have a strong impression on us, Freud devoted a number of pages to the study of dreams pertaining to the death of loved ones. Focusing on the loss of a parent of the opposite sex than that of the dreamer, Freud highlighted the way infantile Oedipal desires remain active in our unconscious. For Freud, the tragic effect of the legend lies in the fulfilment of these childhood wishes which are unacceptable to us as adults and which result in fear and self-punishment.In Lacan's view, Freud limits his reading of *Oedipus* to its manifest content which strips it of any "tragic component" (*SXVII* 113). Whereas Freud took the two crimes committed by Oedipus to constitute the core meaning of the legend, Lacan endeavours to read the Oedipus myth so as to allow its latent content to surface. Lacan's presentation of the Oedipus complex as "Freud's dream" provides a means to achieve this end. Bringing into focus the theme of patricide, Lacan refers to the preface of *The Interpretation of Dreams* where Freud, discussing the mainspring of the book, reflects on the singular experience of losing his father.[1] From here Lacan surmises that "Freud wished to be guilty of his father's murder" (122). To put it in slightly different terms, Freud's elaboration of the Oedipus complex reveals, in a disguised way, his own unconscious desire. The part of the dream which calls for immediate re-interpretation concerns the significance that Freud attributed to the figure of the father.

Alongside the Oedipal myth, Lacan considers the representation of the father in *Totem and Taboo* (1913) where Freud posits the origins of human society and history. The latter is often understood to be a continuation of the Oedipus complex with the origin story providing a historical justification for Freud's theory. Lacan complicates this view by contrasting the role of the father and the meaning of patricide in the two myths. Referring to the origin myth in *Totem and Taboo* as the archetypal "cock-and-bull story", Lacan recalls the constituent elements of the primal horde father who owned all women and denied his sons access (*SXVII* 114).[2] Forced into abstinence the resentful young males decide to murder their father whose position they wished to acquire with the expectation that it would grant access to enjoyment without limit. The murder had the opposite effect. Rather than ensuring their participation in an unlimited pleasure, the guilty sons install the incest prohibition and submit to the law. In this

[1] Commenting on the book's significance, Freud writes: "It was, I found, a portion of my own self-analysis, my reaction to my father's death—that is to say, the most important event, the most poignant loss, of a man's life", p. xxvi.

[2] The theory of the primal horde was first proposed by Charles Darwin in his account of human prehistory when humans lived in large groupings, a primal horde, dominated by one older male who monopolized all females.

way, the power of the dead father is shown to be even greater than that of the living father.

The problem, as Lacan points out, is that "Freud holds this Darwinian buffoonery to be real" (*SXVII* 112). In other words, the "myth" of the primal horde is not exactly a fitting description of the historic significance that Freud attributed to it. Freud believed that the murder of an original father by his jealous sons explained, in fact, the historical origins of the law and of human society whose structure is necessarily patriarchal. Furthermore, the role of the primal father and the consequence of his murder lead to an entirely different outcome than in the Oedipus myth. In the classic Oedipus complex, the law precedes enjoyment and enjoyment takes the form of transgression which comes after the law. As Lacan puts it, if Oedipus does not kill King Laius, then there is no "*jouissance* of the supreme object identified with the mother", Jocasta (122). The tragic level at which Freud appropriates the Oedipal myth, argues Lacan, reveals that "the father's murder is the condition for [*jouissance*]" (120). By contrast, the primal horde myth proceeds along an inverted structure: the father's enjoyment is a basic condition for the establishment of the law (Verhaeghe 2006).[3]

To the extent that Freud understands the father's death to be the result of murder, he limits himself to the view that the father's death is the exclusive consequence of his murder (Van Haute & Geyskens 2016). Lacan interprets the theme of patricide in the Oedipus complex and in *Totem and Taboo* as an attempt on Freud's part to obscure the structural character of the father's castration. Although here, too, there is a crucial difference in Lacan's conceptualization of castration. In Freud's use of the term emphasis is placed on the son's fear of being castrated by the father as punishment for his incestuous desire for the mother. Paul Verhaeghe neatly summarizes that, for Lacan, symbolic castration is "the inevitable consequence of the fact that man becomes a subject and must therefore pass through the signifier in order to gain *jouissance* with the simultaneous implication that *jouissance* is impossible" (2006, 43). Lacan makes use of the equivalence Freud draws between the dead father and

[3] For a detailed comparison between the Oedipal myth and the primal horde myth, see Russell Grigg's "Beyond the Oedipus Complex" pp. 50–68.

enjoyment to signal his own formula of the "real as impossible" (*SXVII* 123). Through reference to the linguistic register of the real, Lacan intends to foreground not the origins of human society and culture, as Freud did, but a structural dimension that falls outside the realm of all possible human meaning.

In place of the almighty patriarch, Lacan introduces the master signifier, <S1>, whose intervention inevitably implies the division of the subject, <$>, and thus castration. Through the use of mathemes, Lacan explains how the same goes for the dead father: "as soon as the father enters the field of the master's discourse [...], he is, from the origins, castrated" (*SXVII* 101). This is precisely what Freud's patricidal theme served to obscure insofar as it presents a defense against the father's castration which concerns his actual limitations. By separating castration from its reference to the murder of the "primal father" and the Oedipus complex, Lacan moves away from the anthropological and pseudo-scientific dimensions of the myth and toward the symbolic function of discourse. For Lacan, castration is "an effect of language" that can only be understood in relation to the chain of signifiers <S1, S2> which are differentially determined (144). Freud's identification with the figure of the father provided a crucial backdrop for Lacan to present his theory of the four discourses in which the father is reduced to being a "structural operator" performing the symbolic agency of the master: castration (123).

While Freud's formulation of the two myths may have masked the image of the castrated father, his case studies paint another picture. In his survey of the latter, Paul Verhaeghe (2006) points to the larger discrepancy that exists between Freud's theory and his clinical work. Alongside mythical representations of strong, prohibiting fathers, Verhaeghe surveys examples from Freud's clinical analyses (the Rat man, the Wolf man, and Little Hans) which illustrate the actuality of sick, weak fathers in need of care (2006, 39–40).[4] Freud's clinical encounter with Dora is especially revealing in this regard.[5] Lacan observes that the entire analysis unfolds from the fact that Dora's father "is strictly a castrated man"

[4] Verhaeghe recalls that "the Rat man lives off his wife's fortunes", the Wolf man wanders around melancholically "from one sanitorium to the next". Verhaeghe also identifies Little Hans "whom Freud urged to assume his Oedipal place despite being a weakling", p. 39.

[5] See *Fragments of an Analysis of a Case of Hysteria* 1900, 1905.

(*SXVII* 95). In addition to being an ill old chap, Lacan stresses the significance Dora attached to the father's sexual impotence. To see the father in this deficient way is to give him what Lacan calls a "symbolic affectation" to measure him against (95). Even after becoming "impotent", Lacan claims that the father retains the title of an "ex-soldier", an "ex-sire" (95). Despite being decommissioned or out-of-action, he continues to carry reference to the possibility of procreation. This symbolic position is at the origin of the father's idealization which is necessary to elevate him to the level of Master.

Lacan raises the function of the idealized father in order not to lose sight of something that Freud "covers [up] with his prejudices" (*SXVII* 94). Throughout *Fragments of an Analysis of a Case of Hysteria*, Freud tried to get Dora to acknowledge her desire for Herr K., her father's substitute. By searching for an archetypically male object to satisfy the hysterical patient's desire, Freud positions himself in relation to Dora as a master, albeit one who fails. Not only did Freud delegitimize Dora's homosexual ties with Frau K., but his use of the Oedipal myth bypassed the question of the hysteric's desire by directing it toward her father. For his part, Lacan underscores the hysteric's "promotion of unsatisfied desire" (74). If the hysteric's desire is a desire that aims at remaining unfulfilled, then Freud's repeated attempts to find a specific object are all doomed to fail. By refusing to acknowledge the notion of a "castrated master", Grigg argues that the Oedipus complex can be read as something Freud produced in response to hysteria, "a response [...] designed to protect the place of the father".

Another way of articulating the limitations of Freud's Oedipus complex is to consider its inability to account for the relationship between the Hysteric and the Master figure. In developing this perspective, Lacan evokes the example of Oedipus as a specific incarnation of the master. Setting aside the myth's manifest content, Lacan puts the accent on Oedipus' encounter with the Sphinx and, by extension, the citizens of Thebes. According to Lacan, Oedipus becomes king by means of "the fact that he has delivered the people from a question decimating its best by seeking to answer what presents itself as an enigma" (*SXVII* 120). Oedipus is above all someone who mastered the Sphinx's test of truth with his knowledge for the sake of protecting the community against danger.

Indicated in Oedipus' response to the riddle is the implication that knowledge and truth are one in the same; there is no separation between the chain of signifiers and the truth they express. As the tragedy unfolds however Oedipus' answer is shown to fall into "the trap of truth" (120). After realizing that he is responsible for his predecessor's murder, Oedipus executes on himself the sentence he pronounced for the murderer. Lacan interprets Oedipus' decision to gouge out his own eyes as an act symbolic of castration. To be castrated constitutes the essence of the Master's position.

Through his discussion on Dora, Lacan replaces the figure of the murdered father with that of the castrated master. Lacan's notion of symbolic castration derives from the differential aspect of signifiers which only signify in reference to other signifiers, thwarting the possibility for truth and knowledge to coincide completely. Every bit of knowledge leaves a remainder. No-one, not even Oedipus, can fully articulate truth for, as Lacan argues, "truth can only be figured through being stated in a half-saying" (*SXVII* 104). This is what the hysteric's desire and the Sphinx's riddle make painfully clear. Lacan observes that the mythical representation of the enigma is supported by the ambiguous being of the Sphinx "in whom a double disposition is incarnated by virtue of being made, like the half-saying, from two half bodies" (*SXVII* 120). Differently put, the Sphinx, like the hysteric, embodies the truth of the castrated master. This is where Freud's "father complex" errs. In his critique of the Freudian perspective, Lacan states:

> Freud's experience with the hysteric, if not for her sayings, at least the configurations she presented him with, should have guided him better here than the Oedipus complex does and led him to consider that [...] at the level of analysis itself, everything is to be put back into question concerning what is necessary from knowledge in order for this knowledge to be called into question in the site of truth. (101)

The hysteric is someone who pursues knowledge for the sake of truth. The truth she incarnates is shown to be structurally lacking and defective like the Master she appoints to solve her enigma. In her promotion of unsatisfied desire, the hysteric stages the scene of truth time and time again in search of a Master. Rising to the challenge, Freud behaved like a master whose shortcomings Dora put on display. Uninterested in the sexual organ Freud's theory had to offer, Dora obtained enjoyment from posing the insoluble question of her identity as a woman.

4.2.2 The Power-Knowledge Nexus

Lacan was not alone in his critique of Freud's Oedipal problematic; Foucault, too, took up the theme on several occasions with the aim of recasting it in a completely new light. Foucault's earliest engagement with Sophocles' tragedy, *Oedipus Rex*, is preserved in the twelfth lecture of the 1970–1971 Collège course *The Will to Know*. Written in the summer of 1972, Foucault delivered a lecture titled "Oedipal Knowledge" (*Le Savoir d'Œdipe*) at the State University of New York and then at Cornell University the same year, which he repeated at the Pontifical Catholic University in Rio de Janeiro in 1974.[6] The latter, known as "Truth and Juridical Forms", deepens the perspectives of the preceding lectures to put forth an account of the Oedipus complex that operated "not at the individual level but at the collective level; not in connection with desire and the unconscious but in connection with power and knowledge" (*TJF* 16). In particular, Foucault was interested in how the Oedipus story could recount the history of a political power erected around the distant historical personage of the Assyrian king.

Drawing on the work of his mentor, Georges Dumézil, Foucault refers to the societal functions of early Indo-European cultures to interpret the drama of Oedipus as enacting the fall of the rule of the early Greek "tyrant", a western offshoot of the Assyrian model of kingship.[7] Foucault's aim is to demonstrate how this archaic model, which linked together a form of knowledge and the function of a political power, was gradually dismantled at the origin of the Greek age of the fifth century. Sophocles'

[6] According to Daniel Defert, there are a total of seven different versions of the lecture in the Foucault archive, p. 279.

[7] See Georges Dumézil, *Jupiter, Mars, Quirinus: essai sur la conception Indo-Européenne de la société sur les origines de Rome* (Paris: Gallimard, 1941); *Mythe et épopée*, vol. 1: *L'Idéologie des trois fonctions dans les épopées des peuples Indo-Européens* (Paris: Gallimard, 1968).

tragedy, argues Foucault, represents the historic dawn of this dismantling; it tells the story of "what had to disappear with classical Greece for its society to exist" (*FS* 32). Situated in a historical dimension, Foucault shifts the Freudian emphasis away from "Oedipus the Incestuous" or "Oedipus the Parricidal" and toward "Oedipus the Tyrant", the professional of political power who existed in the Athenian society of Sophocles' era. From this perspective, Foucault's reading is closer to that of Pierre Vidal Naquet and Jean-Pierre Vernant who, in their essay "Oedipus Without the Complex", write:

> The material of the tragedy is not the dream, postulated as a human reality outside history, but the social thought peculiar to the fifth-century city, with all the tensions and contradictions that appear in it when the advent of law and the institutions of political life place in question the old religious and moral traditional values. (1990, 88)[8]

Foucault's interest in archaic Greece can be further specified in that it reflects a definite positioning within the heritage of Nietzsche, a thinker who transformed western thought by rejecting the founding Greek disjunction between knowledge and power.[9] By foregrounding the status of the tyrant as constitutive of "Oedipal knowledge", Foucault evokes the historical figure of the "expert king" (*roi savant*), man of *technē* or of *gnome*, in whom knowledge and power are entirely correlative, reciprocal, and superimposed. In pre-democratic Greece the term "tyrant" designated an adventurer who, subject to trials of fate, accedes to the throne by virtue of his knowledge rather than justice. After reaching the highest threshold of power, the tyrant is always under threat of losing it. With tyrannical power at stake in Sophocles' tragedy, Foucault presents the Oedipal theme in its historical links to the problem of kingship and the preservation of sovereignty. What gets played out in the Oedipus story, claims Foucault, is "the struggle between kinds of knowledge (*savoir*) and

---

[8] This essay was originally published in 1966.

[9] The belief that knowledge is found in an autonomous pure truth is a myth which Nietzsche dispelled; what lurks behind all knowledge is a struggle for power. See the discussion in Chap. 2: "The Outside of Knowledge".

kinds of power, a struggle between forms of power-knowledge" (*LWTK* 256).

In addition to the Freudian perspective, Foucault's interpretation of *Oedipus* targets the occultation of the history of power by the pre-Nietzschean philosophical tradition. The reference to Sophocles' play can be read, in a methodological sense, as a way of bringing to light (or rather into sight) certain procedures of power which remain otherwise hidden. In a chapter of the book, *Foucault's Theatres*, Kelina Gotman describes how the frame and framework of "seeing" depends on an entire theatrical machinery in order for the representation of power to enact the coming into and out of being of power (2020, 69). Foucault stages the rise of Athenian democracy and the fall of the Greek tyrant against the backdrop of one of the most important processes in the history of the production of truth in the west. Assigning it a proper gravitas in the "course context" of "The Will to Know", Daniel Defert writes that Foucault's lecture "Oedipal Knowledge" plays "something like the role played by *Las Meninas* in relation to the theory of representation in *The Order of Things*" (2013, 279). Foucault later clarified:

> I will speak of the Oedipus story not as a point of origin, as the moment of formulation of man's desire or forms of desire, but, on the contrary, as a rather curious episode in the history of knowledge and as a point of emergence of the inquiry. (*FS* 5)

Foucault's reading of *Oedipus Tyrannos* pieces together the constitutive elements of the transformation of procedures for establishing truth, from the juridico-religious "truth-test" in archaic Greece to the politico-juridical "truth-report" in classical Greece (*LWTK* 279). Foucault describes the archaic practice of producing juridical truth as a "testing game"; a type of challenge hurled by one adversary at another. This way of establishing truth, which does not depend on an investigation, a witness, or an inquiry, disappears with classical Greece. The specificity with which Foucault presents the Oedipal story targets a liminal space of this disappearance. On one hand, the search for truth by Oedipus and the entire city of Thebes marks the point of emergence of the judicial inquiry. On the other hand, remnants of the old truth-test can still be observed in

Sophocles' tragedy. Foucault considers two examples in this regard. Given in the form of a riddle, the first concerns Oedipus' famous encounter with the Sphinx. The second follows from a dispute that occurs between Oedipus and Creon. In response to an accusation Creon challenges Oedipus to swear an oath which precipitates his eventual demise.

The dramatic effect of the play derives from the transformation of the relationships of power and truth; the script, as well as its sequence of events, work to establish new relationships between the two successors to the Theban throne. Monique David-Ménard explains that Oedipus and his brother-in-law, Creon, eventually confront each other politically and in terms of a factual truth: "the power of both is now dependent on the establishment of certain facts" (2010, 25). According to Foucault, the different stages of the inquiry and the facts it gradually discovers follow one another "according to the ritual form and political-religious mechanism of the sumbolon" (*LWTK* 237). Foucault refers to the sumbolon, whose form is dominant throughout *Oedipus the King*, as "the law of halves": the halves that come to complement each other are like "a symbol whose reunited totality has the value of proof and attestation" (234).

In its symbolic dimensions, *Oedipus* is a story of circulating fragments which pass from hand to hand: "from Phoebus to the seer, from Jocasta to Oedipus, from the messenger to the shepherd" (*LWTK* 234). The entire procedure of the search for truth follows the dictates of the sumbolon which enable the "narrative half" to be joined with the "oracle half", the "incest half" with the "murderer half", and the "Theban half" with "Corinthian half" (235). For the sumbolon to be complete, the different pieces of truth must pass from the gods to the kings and from the kings to the slaves. Foucault highlights this trajectory to explain the shift from a prophetic and prescriptive enunciation of the truth to a retrospective statement which is no longer characterised by the magico-religious gaze of prophets, but by the empirical everyday gaze of shepherds. This is the trap that Oedipus unintentionally sets for himself; the sovereign who wanted to see with his own eyes, finds himself guilty in the eyes of witnesses. As a result, Foucault explains that "the sumbolon, which was linked to religious practices, to the exercise of power, [is] now preserved in the new political and social organization of the city" (254).

After Oedipus uses his power as tyrant to pull together the pieces of truth, there is no longer any need for him in the production of the sumbolon. To put it in historical terms, the union between knowledge and power that Oedipus represented falls into disuse at the dawn of Greek democracy. Foucault argues that the power of Oedipus is destroyed because two types of knowledge are fitted together: oracular knowledge and knowledge of the inquiry (*LWTK* 244). As an emblem of power, the sumbolon ensures "two ways of submitting to two socially, politically, and religiously different rituals of knowledge" (254). Through the interplay of the missing halves, the mechanism of the sumbolon turns Oedipus into an excessive figure: "the speeches uttered by Oedipus or concerning Oedipus appear double, as saying two things at the same time" (236). I understand this as a particularly salient point because, contrasted with the Freudian account of Oedipus as a blazon of the unconscious, Foucault provides a portrait of the sovereign who is the bearer of a surplus knowledge, a man of transgression whom the god's oracles and the city's testimonies drive out:

> Everything concerning and around Oedipus is too much: too many parents, too many marriages, fathers who are also brothers, daughters who are also sisters, and this man, so excessively given to misfortune, [...] ought to be tossed into the sea. (257)

In her reading, Gotman explains that the theatrical process of making visible is fundamentally partial: "there is no power where there is not anti-Oedipus" (2020, 69). Gotman locates the image of anti-Oedipus in Foucault's description of the composite figure of the excessive: "that which reminds us that what appears always already powerful contains within it a secret space of undoing, a zone of indeterminacy" (72). With *Oedipus*, Foucault reveals an institution of power that goes beyond the sovereign king, and which the sovereign only temporarily safeguards. The gnomic knowledge which Oedipus engaged to seize the Theban throne eventually came to define political power as a bureaucratic procedure of veridiction. The play's anti-Oedipal forces manifest the powerlessness that is constitutive of power. It demonstrates how power takes place despite the sovereign ruler who is shown to have no sovereignty at all: as soon as Oedipus is ruled upon by the judicial inquiry, he is doomed.

There is also a decidedly Nietzschean dimension to all of this. While traditional Greek philosophy affirms the permanent possibility of an external challenge to power in the name of truth, it leaves out an important episode in the history of truth which Foucault's reading of *Oedipus* throws into relief. Following the major political organization and distribution at the origin of Greek society, Foucault observes that a "fictitious place was fixed where power is founded on a truth" which is subject to a double condition (*LWTK* 193). To be qualified to hold a discourse of truth classical Greek law imposed an ethic of "purity, innocence and non-criminality" while also situating the speaking subject "outside the actual exercise of power" (193). For Foucault, this is the Oedipal constraint that needs to be overturned in the west.

4.3 Read my Desire ... as a Testing Game

In this section, I return to the question raised in Chap. 1 regarding Foucault's relation to desire in the early to mid-1970s. Rather than analyzing what Foucault explicitly says about desire, I choose to focus on the way in which his genealogies can be read as vehicles for expressions of hysterical desire. In developing this perspective, I draw inspiration from the figure of the Sphinx. In the previous Sect. 4.1, the role played the Sphinx was shown to present a test of knowledge to Oedipus. In this section, I develop a perspective in which Foucault's genealogies challenge the discourses of mastery (e.g., philosophical, juridical, and scientific) through the "testing game" which he discusses in "Truth and Juridical Forms" (1974).

To account for the framework of the testing game, I first shift my focus to Foucault's lecture course "Society Must be Defended" (1975–1976). In this course Foucault presents the genealogical use of history not only as a means of reporting struggle, but also as a political tool and weapon in ongoing struggles. I identify Foucault's interest in the "historico-political discourse of war" as a prime example. In conjunction, I consider the significance Foucault attributes to the thematic of war. First, it offers a point of reference for the analysis of power as a multiplicity of relations of force rather than being held concretely by a sovereign. Second and relatedly, I maintain that the binary structure of war derives from a pre-judicial system of challenge and test in which we find the old formula of the duel between two warriors.

4.3.1 Recourse to Ancient Rights

In his lecture course "Society Must Be Defended" (1975–1976) Foucault presents a historical critique of sovereignty as it has been understood in the discourse of political theory and history in the west. One of Foucault's principle targets is the Hobbesian system of power which emanates from a single center: "we have to study power outside the model of the *Leviathan*, outside the field delineated by juridical sovereignty, and the institution of the State" (*SMD* 34). Previously Foucault had examined the power at work in administrative and Statist techniques used in the institutional confinement of "dangerous" individuals (*History of Madness*, 1961). Returning to the problem of power in his lectures at the Collège de France in the early to mid-1970s, Foucault devoted several historical analyses to: (1) the production of truth in ancient Greece, (2) punitive mechanisms used in Europe during the Middle Ages, and (3) the normalizing apparatuses of the disciplinary society. Informed by a trajectory which questions the "how" of power, Foucault now insists that:

> Rather than looking for the single form or the central point from which all forms of power derive, either by way of consequence or development, we must begin by letting them operate in their multiplicity, their differences, their specificity, and their reversibility; we must therefore study them as relations of force that intersect, refer to one another, converge, or, on the contrary, come into conflict and strive to negate one another. (*SMD* 265–66)

According to Foucault, until the seventeenth century theories of power in western political thought were theories of a singular, typically royal, sovereignty. For this reason, history had been erected around the figure of the sovereign. The role of history was to "produce a justification of power and a reinforcement of that power" (*SMD* 66). When deployed in the dimension and function of sovereignty, history established a memorialized continuity of power deriving from ancient kingdoms and heroic kings. Traditional history, claims Foucault, manifested the "great long jurisprudence of a power that has always retained its rights"; it attested to power's place and affirmed that power has always been where it is now (73). The purpose of recounting the history of monarchs and their deeds, argues Foucault, was "to establish a juridical link" between power and its workings which demonstrated, in turn, "the continuity of the law itself" (66). Like funerals and coronations, history was a ritual inherent in the exercise of sovereignty; it intensified power by speaking of right and the luster of glory.

In the sixteenth century, the appearance of a new form of history began to pose a direct challenge to that of sovereignty and kings. Foucault characterizes the emergent discourse as a "counter-history" to the extent that, in it, the function of memory acquires a completely new meaning. Rather than preserving the law by ensuring that power is not forgotten, the task of counter-history is to demystify power's secrets, "to disinter something that has been hidden" out of neglect and deliberate misrepresentation (72). Counter-history disturbs the dazzling effect of power that magnified the glory of the sovereign by revealing the Janus-faced reality of the law: "the triumph of some means the submission of others" (70). Born out of the contingency and injustice of battles, the role of counter-history is to show that "laws deceive, that kings wear masks, that power creates illusions, and that historians tell lies" (72). No longer bound up with the ternary organization or pyramidal description of the social body, Foucault states that counter-history is based on a binary perception and division of society:

> Them and us, the unjust and the just, the masters and those who must obey them, the rich and the poor, the mighty and those who have to work in order to live, those who invade lands and those who tremble before them. (74)

Foucault's critique of sovereignty in "Society Must Be Defended" (1975–1976) finds support in the discourse of "race war" or "race struggle" (*SMD* 63). The term "race", as it functioned in counter-history, is not taken in a literal or even quasi-biological sense.[10] Foucault explains that race originally referred to something of the order of "class" and was, in fact, the discourse from which Marx and Engels founded the concept of "class struggle".[11] This caveat notwithstanding, Foucault's praise for the discourse of "race war" warrants further explanation given the tendency towards racialized violence that marks his substantive discussions on biopolitics. To see what he is after, it is important to recall that Foucault's goal in this lecture course is to investigate the sources, limits, and fecundity of analyzing power in terms of war and military tactics. The organization of war provided a new social physics of power and resistance with forces moving relationally rather then held concretely by a sovereign. For Foucault, the discourse of "race war" rendered power intelligible in the strategic form and warlike logic of struggle rather than the juridical form and regulated or codified logic of rights and sovereignty.

Foucault's interest in war as an analyzer of power relations is evident in his book publications which situate the 1976 course chronologically between *Discipline and Punish* (1975) and the first volume of the History *Sexuality*: La volonté de savoir (1976). The model of war provided an alternative to the economic analysis of power in Marxian discourse and the negative schema of repression in traditional psychoanalytic theory. In celebration of what appears to be a Nietzschean Leftist militant ideal, Foucault's opening lectures set out to test the validity of analyzing power under the rubric of a multiplicity of force relations manifest in a perpetual and underlying war. This hypothesis is initially captured in Foucault's inversion of Carl von Clausewitz's famous aphorism: "war is the continuation of politics by other means" (*SMD* 15). A crucial proviso for understanding

[10] Foucault employs the word "race" to designate a certain historico-political divide: "Two races can be said to exist whenever one writes the history of two groups which do not, initially have the same language or religion [...] The only link between them is the violence of war and its effects: the differences, dissymmetries and barriers created by privileges, customs, rights, distribution of wealth and exercise of power", p. 77.

[11] Foucault insists that "it should not be forgotten that toward the end of his life, Marx told Engels in a letter written in 1882 that 'You know very well where we found our idea of class struggle; we found it in the work of the French historians who talked about the race struggle'", p. 79.

"Society Must Be Defended" is that Foucault does not invert Clausewitz; he claims to identify a counter-historical discourse of "politics as war" which predates Clausewitz's formula. Foucault's way of showing the hypothesis of war at work is to undertake a genealogy of its alleged proponents including the English political theorist, Thomas Hobbes.

In its commentary on Hobbes' *Leviathan*, "Society Must be Defended" marks a vital if not emblematic entry into the problem of sovereignty and the way political authority is established through rights and contracts in the modern liberal tradition. Written during the English Civil War (1642–1651) the *Leviathan* (1651) builds on Hobbes' earlier work *De Cive* (1642) concerning the brute situation of a state of nature, "the war of all against each", used to depict the hypothetical life of people before the organization of societies and the constitution of the State. Understood as a basic and primal situation in which living individuals devour one another, the *Leviathan* represents a key historical reference for examining the function of war in political thought. At first blush Foucault writes that "Hobbes appears to be the man who said that war is both the basis of power relations and the principle that explains them" (*SMD* 89).

Several pages later Foucault inverts this perspective arguing that "Hobbes wanted to eliminate the historical reality of war, as though he wanted to eliminate the genesis of sovereignty" a story which tells not only of victory and triumph but of brutal defeat and bloody conquest (2003, 97). Throwing into relief the theoretical savagery posited by Hobbes, Foucault challenges its primary characteristics: "there are no battles in Hobbes' primitive war, there is no blood and there are no corpses" (92). In place of war, Foucault observes "a field of primal diplomacy" which allows every man to calculate the threat posed by other men's willingness to fight, and to assess the potential risk of entering battle (93). The "clash" of forces occurs indirectly in what Foucault calls a play of presentations; a theatre in which there are "wiles, deceitful expressions", "intentions disguised as their opposite, and worries disguised as certainties" (93).

Foucault understands the elimination of war in contextually specific terms: "the enemy discourse that Hobbes is addressing is the discourse that could be heard in the civil struggles that were tearing the State apart in England" (99). It was a discourse which spoke of dark servitude and forfeiture in which the voices of the defeated could be heard challenging the victors: "we may well have been conquered, but we will not remain conquered" (99). The *Leviathan*'s strategic opposite number, claims Foucault, "is the political use that was being made of historical knowledge" pertaining to struggles that go on beneath the laws and institutions that apparently regulate power (98). Foucault points to the cessation of war in the discourse of rights and contracts to foreground Hobbes' formulation of a relationship of sovereignty: "once the defeated have shown a preference for life and obedience, they make their victors their representatives and restore a sovereign" (95). Foucault points to the way power is dissolved of the element of domination whenever it is masked by the "legitimate rights of the sovereign" on one hand, and "the legal obligation to obey", on the other hand (26).

Rather than analyzing the exercise of power from the standpoint of the sovereign, Foucault focused his approach on the extremities and outer limits, "the point where [power] becomes capillary" (*SMD* 27). Through the lens of a history of dominations Foucault sought to grasp the "material agency of subjugation" by discovering how multiple bodies, forces, energies, and thoughts are progressively constituted as subjects (28). The invention of a new mechanics of discipline in the seventeenth and eighteenth centuries revealed that power depended on a tight grid of material coercions and constant surveillance for its operation which could no longer be transcribed in terms of relations of sovereignty. Despite the change in power's functioning, Foucault explains that the theory of sovereignty continued to organize the juridical codes in Europe; it served as a "critical instrument" against the monarchy and made it possible "to superimpose a system of right" on disciplinary power which concealed its mechanism and erased from it the technique of domination (37). The gradual democratization of sovereignty and the establishment of a public right, argues Foucault, resulted in a circular gridlock whereby:

> [T]he only existing and apparently solid recourse we have against the usurpations of disciplinary mechanics […] is precisely a recourse or a return to a right that is organized around sovereignty […] we should not be turning to the old right of sovereignty; we should be looking for a new right that is

> both anti-disciplinary and emancipated from the principle of sovereignty. (39–40)

One way of grasping Foucault's interest in the thematic of war is to consider how it intersects with a right that is at once new and ancient. "New" in the sense that it represents a strategic resurgence of the occultation of the history of power by traditional historians and philosophers alike. "Ancient" in the sense that it derives from a pre-judicial system of challenge and test. Such a right forms the backdrop of Foucault's version of *Oedipus the King*; a story which narrates the fall of the sovereign by a structure of power in which agency is held marginally in the extremities of public life. Far removed from traditional history which seeks to preserve the uninterrupted nature of the genealogy of kings and their power, Foucault's reading of *Oedipus* revolves around a basic discontinuity which distinguishes features of archaic Greek society from the system of classical Greek law. Within this liminal space, I argue that Foucault establishes recourse to remnants of a right in the form of a "testing game" whose binary structure evokes the formula of a duel; a tête-à-tête contest arranged between two warriors who circumvent the insertion of a political authority who would function above their heads as law.

4.3.2 Truth in the Discourse of War

There are at least two historical examples of the "testing game" mentioned by Foucault. The first, discussed in his lectures on "The Will to Know" (1970–1971), is the magico-religious test of the oath which renders the formulation of truth visible within a system of struggle. Given in the form of a "truth-challenge", the ritual procedures of the test were put to work by private individuals seeking to settle a dispute outside the juridical apparatus offered by the organization of the State (2013, 78). Foucault emphasizes that the game of the test worked without truth having to manifest itself; it was indicated indirectly through a gesture, the oath, and the person who swore it. Once the challenge was accepted, the oath shifted the combat into another universe dominated by the power of the gods where the risks were "incommensurable with those of the struggle" and governed by laws "hidden from human sight" (77). Contrary, however, to the system of law in classical Greece where truth is invited to come out in the tribunal domain, that is, in the already constituted space of sovereignty, Foucault explains that:

> In pre-law, between two adversaries who accept neither the sovereignty of one in relation to the other nor a sovereignty exercised over both, the test of truth appeals to an unlimited and wild sovereignty. (78)

A second example can be observed in "Truth and Juridical Forms" (1974) where Foucault discusses "the feudal judicial test" in ancient Germanic law.[12] Like the archaic practice of the truth-challenge, feudal law of the Germanic type settled disputes among individuals according to the system of the test. In addition to the social, verbal, and oath-swearing tests, Foucault recounts a scene from the Carolingian Empire in which accused persons were subjected to rigorous corporal tests known as "ordeals" (2000, 38). The physical test, whether it entailed walking barefoot on burning coal or being bound by rope and submerged in water, transposed the struggle between adversaries onto a confrontation of the individual body with the natural elements. With the tribunal space functioning as an arena for combat, the judicial test was a way of proving not the truth but "the strength, weight, and importance" of the person who passed it (37). In cases where two parties of a disagreement consented to battle, a representative of political authority would intervene only to attest to the regularity of the procedure to verify that the fight went according to the rules. In summary, Foucault states that:

> The judicial test was a way of ritualizing war or of transposing it symbolically. It was a way of giving it a certain number of secondary, theatrical forms, so that the stronger would be designated thereby as the one who was right. (2000, 39)

These examples highlight a crucial aspect of Foucault's appeal for the schema of war in "Society Must Be Defended" (1975–1976). Distinct

[12] See Michel Foucault, *Power* (Essential Works Vol. 3), New York: New Press, 2000.

from elements of the judicial inquiry, the test of truth involves a trial of strength in which weapons are the final judges. The system of the test can be situated in opposition to a tradition of modern thought which has its roots in a constituent element of Greek philosophy, namely, "the identification of truth with peace and neutrality" (2003, 52). The focal point of Foucault's interest in the discourse of war, as it emerged in England, and later in France, is that it forces the historian "to take sides and to abandon the median position of referee, judge, or universal witness" which jurists and philosophers, from Hobbes to Kant, had dreamed of occupying (283). Grounded in history and decentered from a juridical sovereignty, the discourse of war recognizes the normative landscape of the political as something which can only be shaped through one's investment in a struggle. Crucial for understanding this point is the conception of truth at work in "historico-political" discourse, which is fundamentally partial, that is, reserved for partisans. As Foucault put it:

> [I]f the subject who speaks of right (or rather, of rights) is speaking the truth, that truth is no longer the universal truth of the philosopher. It is true that this discourse about the general war, this discourse that tries to interpret the war beneath peace, is indeed an attempt to describe the battle as a whole and to reconstruct the general course of the war. But that does not make it a totalizing or neutral discourse; it is always a perspectival discourse. It is interested in the totality only to the extent that it can see it in one-sided terms, distort it and see it from its own point of view. (52)

This comment intersects with the principle of sacrifice which Foucault identifies in his article "Nietzsche, Genealogy and History (1971) which foregoes any belief in the neutrality, objectivity, and disinterestedness of the subject of knowledge. In "Society Must be Defended", Foucault takes a step further in that he sees the discourse of war as putting forward a truth that functions as a weapon:

> The truth is, in other words, a truth that can be deployed only from its combat position, from the perspective of the sought for victory and ultimately, so to speak, of the survival of the speaking subject himself. (52)

Foucault takes truth to be a weapon in that it helps constitute the speaking subject as *subject*, as an embodied "we" or "I" engaged in a struggle against objective claims of right and truth. This way of constituting subjects stands opposed to "philosophico-juridical" discourses which labor under the pretension of a pacified universality and takes for its interpretive principle a basic rationality that is permanently linked to the just and good. Historico-political discourse, on the other hand, inverts the "traditional values of intelligibility" by asking the fury of passions to explain the calm and order in society (2003, 54). With war as a cipher for peace, the focus shifts from universal law toward that which is most confused, disorganized, and subject to chance and error; "the obscurity of contingencies and all the minor accidents that bring about defeats and ensure victories" (54). Reason is thus shown to be bound up with fragility and illusion; it represents the cunning and wickedness of those who have won a temporary battle and who seek to preserve the relation of domination through calculations, strategies, and technical procedures. The partisan who proclaims truth from a decentered position, in contrast, accentuates the relationship of force based on "a crude and naked irrationality" (55). By inverting the explanatory axis of law and history, historico-political discourse establishes:

> [A] right that is stamped with dissymmetry and that functions as a privilege that has to be either maintained or re-established … For a subject speaking such a discourse, the universal truth and general right are illusions or traps. (268)

In his article "Power/Knowledge", Joseph Rouse argues that there is a close parallel within epistemology "to the preoccupation of political reflection with sovereignty as Foucault construes it" (2005, 106). Recalling the constituent elements of political sovereignty, Rouse describes a "unitary regime, representing legitimacy through the law, established from an impartial standpoint, above particular conflicts, and enforced through discontinuous interventions that aim to suppress illegitimacy" (106). Although he does not mention it, the structure of power that Rouse describes is depicted in the frontispiece of the *Leviathan* which Foucault criticized in "Society Must Be Defended" by analyzing power on the basis of a multiplicity of force relations manifest in a perpetual war. The point on which Rouse insists is that Foucault has the same dual criticism of the conception of political sovereignty to that which he has of "epistemic sovereignty". Rouse's description of the latter further accentuates the analogy:

> [E]pistemic sovereignty constitutes knowledge as the unified network of truths that can be extracted from the circulation of conflicting statements … they are legitimated as truths by the precepts of the rational method, the epistemic surrogate for law. Yet this legitimation does not produce knowledge in the sense of producing new possibilities for truth. Rather, it allows truth to stand forth by suppressing error and irrationality … those statements which do not conform to the regime it establishes. (106)

Just as sovereign power stands above and adjudicates conflicts among its subject powers, epistemic sovereignty, explains Rouse, "is the standpoint above disputes among competing truth-claims" (106). In the French intellectual context, the aspiration for epistemic sovereignty was designated by the quest for the status of science. Foucault's response to that aspiration is that it overlooks the power-effects inherent in the claim to being a science: "what speaking subject, what discursive subject, what subject of experience and knowledge are you trying to minorize … when you begin to say 'I am a scientist'" (2003, 10). Epistemic sovereignty, in other words, dangerously misconstrues its own positioning; it is the modern nexus of power and knowledge which governs the production of knowing subjects and known truths. Part of what constitutes the element of obscurity is the way the problematic of the Enlightenment has been described by scientific discourse in the nineteenth and twentieth centuries. Foucault stresses the imagery and symbolism at work in these descriptions to show how they conceal a "lower" battleground of forces while giving the appearance that the war has been won:

> The progress of Enlightenment, the struggle of knowledge against ignorance, of reason against chimeras, of experience against prejudices, of reason against error, and so on. All this has been described as, or symbolized

> by, light gradually dispelling darkness, and it is this, I think, that we have to get rid of … we have to see … something very different: an immense and multiple battle, but not one between knowledge and ignorance, but an immense and multiple battle between knowledges in the plural—knowledges that are in conflict because of their very morphology, because they are in the possession of enemies, and because they have intrinsic power-effects. (179)

Prior to the eighteenth century, "science" in the singular did not exist. Contemporary with the application of disciplinary power to bodies, Foucault observed a different form of disciplinarization applied to knowledges, in the plural. The disciplinary policing of heterogenous knowledges and their polymorphous singularity, claims Foucault, gave rise to a new constraint not of truth, but of science (185). The uniform apparatus of the university, which emerged at the same time, played a monopolizing role in the selection of knowledges, meaning that any knowledge that existed in the wild, born outside of its institutional field, was automatically and, from the outset, disqualified *a priori*. The establishment of a well-recognized scientific community organized around a consensus enabled the homogenization of knowledges by arranging them into a hierarchical classification. The State, either directly or indirectly, intervened in the pyramidal centralization of knowledges which allowed their content to be controlled at the level of transmission according to certain overall directions.

The discplinarization of knowledges was not without confrontation. At the end of the eighteenth century, Foucault explains that attempts to establish a State knowledge, an official teaching, made only more visible "the decentered history of subjects in struggle" (186). In the field of historical knowledge, disciplinarization did not occur due to a series of struggles, invasions, and confiscations that strengthened its arsenal of weapons. On the other side of a knowledge that has been disciplinarized, Foucault points to the presence of a historical consciousness that is "polymorphous, combative, and divided" (186). As far as historical knowledge goes back, it only encounters an unending war. War is not something history can escape, look down on from above, discover its basic laws, or impose certain limits on it. This is because "war itself supports this knowledge, runs through this knowledge and determines [it]" (173). In speaking of a historical knowledge of struggles, Foucault echoes the Nietzschean claim that knowledge is always a strategic relation in which man finds himself placed:

> The perspectival character of knowledge does not derive from human nature, but always from the polemical and strategic character of knowledge. One can speak of the perspectival character of knowledge because there is a battle and knowledge is the effect of this battle. (*SMD* xxi)

To arrive at this view, Foucault pursued the methodological path of a "genealogy of knowledges". Unlike the "history of science" which he locates on the "cognition-truth" axis, a genealogy of knowledges is situated on what Foucault calls the "discursive practice-clash of power" axis (178). Compared to the attempt to inscribe knowledge in the hierarchy of science, the work of genealogy consists in playing delegitimized knowledges against the power-effects of established social scientificity. The efficacy of discontinuous and local knowledges derives from their positioning in the wild; they are *sauvage*, untethered to any standpoint of sovereignty. The elements of knowledge which the genealogist digs out of the mud and blood of battles could run the risk of being recoded and recolonized by the unitary discourses which once disqualified and excluded them. In response to the danger that these genealogical fragments might be reannexed by scientific discourse and included in their own power-effects, Foucault says that "we could throw down a challenge and say, 'Just try it!'" (12). When viewed through the thematic of war, Foucault's genealogy of knowledges can be seen as a testing game directed at the University (or scientific) discourse.

4.4 The Binary Structure of the Modern Discursive Arena

In this section I attempt to abandon the standpoint of sovereignty in favor of the binary structure of the "testing game". The objective is to isolate and enable a view of the modern discursive arena as being split between two discourses (e.g., the Hysteric and the University) which mobilize the opposition of two forces: hysterical desire versus perverse drive. To this end, I develop a psychoanalytic register to analyze the strategy and tactics at work in each.

4.4.1 Hysterical Desire Versus Perverse Drive

How might the psychoanalytic "forces" of desire and drive enable us to grasp Foucault's genealogical thematic of constant war? The operations of hysterical desire and perverse drive can be observed in the way each discourse (e.g., Hysteric and University) positions itself in relation to knowledge which allows us to identify a relationship of power. One way of approaching this dynamic is from a clinical perspective. The work of Lacan provides clinicians with three main diagnostic structures which indicate different ways of solving problems of alienation, separation, and of castration or the limits on one's enjoyment. Among these structures are neurosis and perversion. Rather than being descriptive names referring to symptoms, these names represent structural positions that indicate specific ways of navigating the world of language with others. I rely mainly on Bruce Fink's text (1999) *A Clinical Introduction to Lacanian Psychoanalysis: Theory and Technique* in developing an understanding of hysterical desire and perverse drive.

Lacan's formula for perversion <*a* ◊ A> presents a useful starting point in that it can be compared with the formula for hysteria <*a* ◊ Ⱥ> in a way that illustrates the similarities and differences between the pervert and the hysteric. From here we can observe that both the hysteric and the pervert occupy the role of object-cause <*a*> in relation to the Other but do so for completely different ends. The hysteric's strategy, discussed in Chap. 1, involves captivating the Other by presenting herself as desirable object for knowledge while also refusing to be the object that would satisfy the desire she provokes, in order to remain what is at stake.[13] Fink describes the hysteric as the subject who "constitutes herself, not in relation to the erotic object she herself has lost, but as the object the Other is missing"

[13] See discussion in the Sect. 2.3.2 of Chap. 2, "The Riddle of Hysteria".

(1999, 120). Rather than taking the object for herself, the hysteric seeks to divine the Other's desire and to become the object that, when missing, makes the Other desire. The pervert, by contrast, employs a completely different strategy in the role of object cause <*a*> in relation to the Other.

In Seminar XI: *The Four Fundamental Concepts of Psychoanalysis* (1964–1965), Lacan locates the structure of perversion in the interplay between drive and *objet a*, and identifies the pervert as he who situates himself in a particular relation to the drive. The pervert, Lacan claims, "determines himself as object" of the drive for the Other's enjoyment (*SXI* 185). Whereas the hysteric positions herself as the object-cause of the Other's *desire*, the pervert positions himself as the object-cause of the Other's *jouissance*. The pervert believes that what the Other lacks and therefore wants is *jouissance* and strives to make the Other exist through being complete by bringing *jouissance* to the Other. Unlike the hysteric, the pervert seeks out a partner who is, at first, a barred Other, <A̸>, whose lack he seeks to cancel, <A>, by making himself the object-cause of the Other's enjoyment. For Lacan, the pervert is "the subject reconstituted through alienation at the cost of being nothing but the instrument of *jouissance*" (*É* 654). Through his attempts to plug up the lack in the Other, the pervert, an instrument, gains enjoyment.

One similarity between the two structures concerns the way each relate to the fundamental fantasy which Lacan describes as a relationship that the subject has with the *objet a*, written as <$ ◊ *a*>. The hysteric's fantasy involves an Other who is, at first blush, the one who desires in the same way that the pervert's fantasy involves an Other who is, outwardly, one who experiences *jouissance*. Beneath the surface of the fantasy structure, however, lies the fact that both the pervert and the hysteric direct the entire scenario. For her part, the hysteric brings the Other to desire in the manner of her choosing and desires as if she were the Other. In a similar vein, the pervert causes the Other to experience *jouissance* in a manner of his choosing while controlling the *jouissance* he reserves for himself. Unlike the pervert, however, the hysteric seeks a partner who is at first an unbarred Other <A>, whom she then inscribes with lack <A̸> in the form of the Other's desire for her. Refusing to be the instrument of the Other's *jouissance*, hysterical desire introduces the possibility for encountering what Lacan called "the castrated master".

Conversely, Jacques-Alain Miller suggests that "perversion can be spoken of as the fear of the Other's castration" (1996, 317). The pervert wishes to see any lack in the Other as something that can be filled or covered up. In contrast to the hysteric's castrating game which involves sustaining the lack in the Other, the pervert must continuously plug up the holes in the Other's knowledge. Perversion is thus a solution to the problem of castration which involves the mechanism of negation. Lacan claims that the *objet a* in perversion "is the foundation of an identification disavowed by the subject" (*SXI* 186). The subject disavows his or her perverse role; s/he believes himself to be a powerful Other and his victim to be reduced to the status of an object when it is, in fact, the other way around <*a* ◊ A>. By disavowing the lack in the Other, the pervert suffers from an excess of enjoyment and finds relief and control in transferring some of his or her surplus enjoyment to the Other's account perhaps in a manner akin to the structure of the Discourse of the University, as I hope to show in what follows.

Contrary to the hysterical subject who gains a secondary satisfaction from posing her identity in the form of a question, the pervert obtains enjoyment in knowing exactly who he is: 'I am the object that completes the Other'. The pervert's relation to knowledge is that of a "professional", a "savant", or an "expert". Defined as the one who knows, the one who can provide answers when asked, the pervert also has a well-defined and carefully delimited scientific object. When confronted with something that would indicate a lack of knowledge of this object, the pervert immediately covers it up with the extension of already existing paradigms. The pervert may appear in the guise of encyclopedic knowledge or as an abject tool in the hands of a non-lacking Other, whether a political, military, or scientific leader. In her article "The Conformity of Perversion", Kristen Hyldgaard argues that the perverse structure is "conservatory with regard to tradition" (2004).[14] By maintaining the status quo in relation to knowledge and truth, the pervert can only function as a stand-in to fill out holes while supplementing and confirming the new law and order as

[14] Kristen Hyldgaard's article is available at: https://www.lacan.com/conformper.htm. [Accessed 4 June 2020.]

if this order had always been there. In contrast, hysterical desire stands for subversion as such, as Hyldgaard puts it:

> The [hysteric] is the castrator in relation to knowledge […] the neurotic is capable of naming an alien element, an occurrence, or an event necessary for opening a new field of thought.[15]

In his article "Can One Exit the Capitalist Discourse Without Becoming a Saint?" Slavoj Žižek considers the opposition of hysterical desire versus perverse drive—in terms of a forceful interaction between the Hysteric's discourse and University discourse, respectively. On one hand, there is the University logic of domination through knowledge <S2>. The university discourse speaks from the place of a supposedly neutral, scientific, and technical knowledge which excludes any subjective position of enunciation. It functions as a paradigm of authority while camouflaging its power through reason and rationality, presenting what amounts to a political decision as a simple insight into the factual state of things (Žižek 2016; Zupančič 2006). On the other hand, the Hysteric's discourse stands for the notion of subjectivity as a destabilizing force of incessant self-expansion. As an agent of insatiable desire, the hysteric subject is imbued with radical questioning and doubt which undermines the certainty and objectivity claimed by scientific fact. It poses a threat to those who claim to possess mastery over knowledge while revealing the material reality, indeed corporeality, of its power.

I make use of these comments to view the opposing forces of hysterical desire and perverse drive as battling each other on the stage of history. If desire is operative in Foucault's genealogies, as a testing game, it is perhaps activated in response to the way the modern discursive space itself has been produced through the constraint of science. The already constituted field of scientific knowledge necessarily leaves a remainder; it cannot state the whole truth about its object. Rather than being situated on the cognition-truth axis, Foucault's genealogy of knowledges is located on "the discursive-practice clash of power axis", directed at the University discourse (*SMD* 178). The intertwining of the Hysteric and the University

[15] Hyldgaard, *op. cit.*

discourses points to the underlying binary structure of modernity. Moreover, it highlights the precariousness of the battleground on which relations of force are played out. The overlapping element can be observed at the level of the discursive structure. The divided subject <$> is both the agent of the hysteric's discourse and the product of the university. Likewise, knowledge <S2> is the agent of the university and the product of the hysteric's discourse. In progressing to the end of one discourse, we might find ourselves on the other side of the twisted structure of the Möbius band.

4.5 Staging an Exit

This chapter has focused primarily on the thematic of constant war as a way of grasping the genealogical use of history. The clinical perspective discussed in the previous section provided a means to situate Foucault's genealogical critique in a kind of "theatre of war" played out between the opposing forces of hysterical desire and perverse drive which find their support in the structure of fantasy. The significance of war was presented as enabling a point of reference for the analysis of power as a multiplicity of forces. It was also discussed in relation to a binary structure that runs throughout society which inevitably places subjects on one side or the other. The principle of sacrifice was used to explain how the genealogist foregoes the belief in the neutrality, objectivity, and disinterestedness of the subject of knowledge. Truth in historico-political discourse was shown to function as a weapon based on its constitutive partiality. The partial character of truth was linked, on the side of the hysteric, to the claim that truth can only be figured through being a half-saying. In this way, the clash between the Hysteric's and the University discourses demonstrates that truth exists in a circular relationship with systems of power, revealing not static states of domination but a perpetual incitation and struggle.

Chapter 4 also marks the end of Part I "The Hysteric" and reflects on the possibilities, for Foucault, of staging an exit from this discourse and, by extension, from the problematic of war. Implicitly, we can see how Foucault's genealogical critique of "epistemic sovereignty" broaches the political and ethical problems involved in ridding oneself of the master's knowledge and the master's reason. One thinks of Nietzsche in this respect who suffered a severe mental collapse towards the end of his life. Chapters 1–3 made use of the discursive structure of hysteria, rather than a psychiatric diagnosis, as a means of grasping the political significance of Foucault's genealogies. The situation of Foucault's research in the late 1970s and early 1980s enacts a new perspectival shift, one that transforms his positioning, through language, to the critical tradition of Kant and to Enlightenment philosophy more broadly.

References

Breuer, J., & Freud, S. (1974) *Studies on Hysteria*. Harmondsworth: Penguin Books.

David-Ménard, M. (2010) "About Anti-Oedipus". *Recherches en psychanalyse*, 10, pp. 202–212. Available at https://doi.org/10.3917/rep.010.0021 [Accessed 6 October 2019].

Fink, B. (1999) *A Clinical Introduction to Lacanian Psychoanalysis: Theory and Technique*. Massachusetts: Harvard University Press.

Foucault, M. (1976) *Mental Illness and Psychology.* Translated from the French by A. Sheridan. New York: Harper and Row.

Foucault, M. (1977) "Nietzsche, Genealogy, History", in Bouchard, D. F. (ed.) *Language, Counter-memory, Practice: Selected Essays and Interviews*. Ithaca, NY: Cornell University Press, pp. 139–164.

Foucault, M. (1990) *Politics, Philosophy, Culture Interviews and Other Writings 1977 –1984*. Kritzman, L. D. (ed). New York: Routledge.

Foucault, M. (2000) "Truth and Juridical Forms", in Faubion, J. (ed.) *Foucault: Power*. New York: New Press. pp. 31–35.

Foucault, M. (2001) *Fearless Speech*, Pearson, J. (ed.). Translated from the French by J. Pearson. Los Angeles: Semiotext(e).

Foucault, M. (2003) *Society Must Be Defended: Lectures at the Collège de France 1975–1976,* Bertani, M., & Fontana, A. (eds.). Translated from the French by D. Macey. New York: Picador.

Foucault, M.. (2013) *Lectures on the Will to Know: Lectures at the Collège de France 1970–1971*, D. Defert, (ed.). Translated from the French by G. Burchell. Basingstoke: Palgrave Macmillan.

Gotman, K. (2020) "Foucault, Oedipus, Négritude", in Fisher, T., & Gotman, K. (eds.) *Foucault's Theatres*. Manchester: Manchester University Press, pp. 63–81.

Hyldgaard, K. (2004) "The Conformity of Perversion", *Symptom - Journal for Lacan*, 5.

Lacan, J. (1978) *The Seminar of Jacques Lacan, Book XI: The Four Fundamental Concepts of Psychoanalysis*, J. A. Miller (ed.). Translated from the French by A. Sheridan. New York/London: W. W. Norton & Company.

Lacan, J. (2002) *Écrits*. Translated from the French by B. Fink, in collaboration with H. Fink & R. Grigg. New York: W.W. Norton.

Lacan, J. (2007) *The Seminar of Jacques Lacan, Book XVII: The Other Side of Psychoanalysis, 1969–1970,* Miller, J. A. (ed.). Translated from the French by R. Grigg. New York: W.W. Norton and Company.

Miller, J.-A. (1996) "On perversion", in Feldstein, R., Fink, B., & Jaanus, M. (eds.) *Reading Seminars I and II: Lacan's Return to Freud*. Albany: SUNY, pp. 306–320.

Rouse, J. (2005) "Power/Knowledge", in Gutting, G. (ed.) *The Cambridge Companion to Foucault*. Cambridge: Cambridge University Press, pp. 95–122.

Van Haute, P., & Geyskens, T. (2016) "Freud's Dream? Lacan and Oedipus", in TomŠiČ, S., & Zevnik, A. (eds.), *Jacques Lacan between Psychoanalysis and Politics*. London/New York: Routledge, pp. 47–61.

Verhaeghe, P. (2006) "Enjoyment and Impossibility: Lacan's Revision of the Oedipus Complex", in Grigg, R., & Clemens, J. (eds.) *Jacques Lacan and the Other Side of Psychoanalysis: Reflections on Seminar XVII*. Durham: Duke University Press, pp. 29–50.

Žižek, S. (2016) "Can One Exit From the Capitalist Discourse Without Becoming a Saint", *Crisis and Critique*, 3 (3). Available at: http://crisiscritique.org/political11/Slavoj.pdf. [Accessed: 27 January 2021].

———. (2006) "When Surplus Enjoyment Meets Surplus Value", in Grigg, R., & Clemens, J. (eds.) *Jacques Lacan and the Other Side of Psychoanalysis: Reflections on Seminar XVII*. Durham: Duke University Press, pp. 155–178.

Part II

The Analyst's Discourse

5

Le Point de Capiton: Two Kantian Legacies

5.1 Introduction

In Seminar XVII: *The Other Side of Psychoanalysis* (1969–1970), Lacan makes a profound conceptual link between his earlier formulation of the *point de capiton* and the productive function of the master signifier which underpins his theory of the four discourses. Referring to Seminar III: *The Psychoses* (1955–1956), Lacan recalls the imagery of the *point de capiton* to illustrate how "something that spreads throughout language like wildfire is readable […], how it hooks on, creates a discourse" (*SXVII* 189). For Lacan, the "readability" of any text is contingent on finding that which constitutes a master signifier. In this chapter, I draw on Lacan's notion of the *point de capiton* to support my proposition regarding Foucault's discursive passage from the Hysteric to the Analyst. I identify in Foucault's writings the intervention of the signifier in the form of a name as that which both defines the readability and effects a restructuration of the body of texts treated my Part I, "The Hysteric". I argue that Foucault's use of the signifier "Kant" in the late 1970s and early 1980s performs a resignification of the discourses of modernity which enacts a

J. L. Davis, *Reading Foucault Through Lacan*, The Palgrave Lacan Series,
https://doi.org/10.1007/978-3-031-69738-8_5

perspectival shift from the Hysteric's discourse and makes readable his new positioning in the Analyst's discourse.

The claim that Foucault can be read within the Discourse of the Analyst calls for immediate clarification. It is well known that Foucault's work provides a critique of the danger represented by psychoanalysis in the development of a modern disciplinary society.[1] Foucault's concerns about psychoanalysis are linked to his overall aim to expose the dangers involved in what is taken as self-evident, universal, and necessary. To detach from the perspective according to which psychoanalytic thought is simply another power-knowledge regime that produces subjects as subjected beings, I rely on Lacan's definition of the Analyst's discourse in Seminar XVII. Lacan carefully separates the "psychoanalyzing discourse" from that of the Analyst, claiming that "what the analyst establishes as analytic experience is the structural introduction, under artificial conditions, of the Hysteric's discourse" (*SXVII* 33). The Discourse of the Analyst, in other words, unfolds through that of the Hysteric on which it remains structurally dependent. In Part I, I presented Foucault's "hystorical critique", with emphasis on "the genealogy of knowledges", in its discursive capacity to question and combat the singular, contingent, and arbitrary constraints of scientific modernity.

In this chapter, I focus on the conceptual landscape that Lacan develops to give a new rigor to the psychoanalytic account of language. Section 5.2.1, "From a Theory of the Sign to Discourse Theory", outlines Lacan's attempts to reinscribe the Freudian enterprise and to bring into focus its thoroughly linguistic character. This is especially evident in Lacan's essay "The Agency of the Letter in the Unconscious" (1957) in which the Swiss linguist Ferdinand de Saussure appears as his primary theoretical support. I provide an overview of Lacan's inventive re-working of Saussurean diction to introduce Lacan's concepts of the "signifying chain", the "signifier", and the "signified". With these terms, Lacan accounts for the differential relation of symbolic elements and their articulations which show how the production of meaning is contingent upon a particular relationship of signifiers. I present Lacan's theory of the signifier as

[1] See *The History of Sexuality*, Vol. 1, p. 21.

forging a crucial step toward his conceptualization of discourse in Seminar XVII.

In Sect. 5.2.2, "Enter the Analyst", I discuss the changes in Lacan's understanding of language in terms of a theoretical shift from a structuralist conception of a "closed order" of signifiers to a discursive relation of signifiers that always produce a signifying remainder, symbolized as <*a*>. This allows us to grasp Lacan's symbolic order in its constitutive incompleteness which maintains the illusion of its consistency through a set of exclusions. I explore how the re-inscription of the excluded term by the Discourse of the Analyst changes the previously closed order of symbolic elements through the production of a new signifying chain. I introduce Lacan's notion of the *point de capiton* (or "nodal point" in discourse theory) to show how he accounts for the partial fixation of meaning; the point at which the signifier and the signified are stitched together in a signifying chain, albeit temporarily. The concept of discursive formations regulated by *points de capiton* recognizes both the impossibility of structural closure and the inevitability of surplus meaning that escapes final fixation.

I present this discussion under the Sect. 5.2 heading "Between Reality and the Real". On the one hand, Lacan's concept of discourse describes the reality that underpins the world in which we live or at least the one we know. Lacan's description of the symbolic order as a network of differential relations among signifying elements provides a basis for understanding the categories and identities through which subjectivity and social reality are produced. On the other hand, if the symbolic order does not represent a structural totality, then it cannot completely fix social identity (nor can it fully symbolize bodily enjoyment). This opens the space for language to take a new form that might consist in something other than the illusory projection of closure, fullness, and self-transparency of the subject onto a particular content. With Lacan's formula of the Real as an impossible plenitude in Seminar XVII, I link the production of the master signifier in the Analyst's discourse with the possibility of signifying a new relation to the Real.

Section 5.3, "A Retroactive Constitution of Meaning", applies Lacan's notion of the *point de capiton*, and the related concept of the "signifying chain", to account for Foucault's passage from the Hysteric's discourse to the Analyst's discourse. I draw on Lacan's graph of the elementary cell of desire to highlight the suturing movement of the *point de capiton* which stabilizes a group of floating signifiers by partially fixing their meaning. Prior to the *capitonnage* the signifiers can be arranged in a way that reflects the uncertain meaning of a half-finished sentence. Signifiers do not signify until they are tied to a signified through the retroactive effect of the chain's punctuation. Stressing the dual temporality of retroaction and anticipation that structures the process of signification, I consider Foucault's late and early writings on Kant. In Section 5.3.1, "The Kantian Division Revisited", I discuss how, for Foucault, the identificatory signifier "Kant" has a shifting and contingent signified with no stable referent. I claim that, from its inception, Foucault's signifying chain lacks punctuation.

Section 5.3.2, "Tutelage and the Way Out", attempts to isolate the moment of the *point de capiton* in which Foucault constitutes the previously floating signifiers as a meaningful chain. I identify Foucault's lecture course "The Government of Self and Others" (1982–1983) as the site of the retroactive determination of meaning. In the opening lectures of this course, Foucault distinguishes between two Kantian legacies and establishes a relationship between Kant's *Critique* and his later response to the question of *Aufklärung*. I argue that these two elements effect a restructuration of the past contingent traces of the signifier "Kant" through the discursive structure of the Analyst which produces a new signifying chain. I explain the movement of the *point de capiton* along the lines of the movement of metaphor which concerns the moment the signifier crosses the bar and reveals the signification of the term "Kant". Bearing in mind Lacan's critique of a structural totality, I present my reading of Foucault as imposing a partial, temporary closure which leaves open the space for the next new meaning.

Chapter 5 marks a significant albeit unexpected contribution to the growing body of interpretive literature concerning Foucault's relation to Kant's critical philosophy (Han 2002; Allen 2008; Koopman 2010). In a field dominated by "Foucauldian" scholars, debates over Foucault's connection to Kant risk being read through the lens of a closed order of signifiers that only signify in relation to each other. By drawing Lacanian theory into these discussions, I hope to reflect the outside of contemporary thinking on the matter in order to explore what new knowledges can be read.

5.2 Between Reality and the Real

Lacan's account of discourse, as formulated in Seminar XVII (1969–1970), captures the theoretical shifts and ambiguities of his earlier work. In Sect. 5.2.1, "From a Theory of the Sign to Discourse Theory", I discuss Lacan's initial understanding of language as a "closed order of signifiers" that operate according to a system of differential couplings. This is evident in Lacan's essay (1957) "The Agency of the Letter in the Unconscious" in which he attempts to fuse Freud's theory with Saussurean linguistics. In this essay, Lacan transposes Ferdinand de Saussure's structuralist theory of the sign to the psychoanalytic field which produces another and different model of the linguistic process.[2] I explain how Lacan converts Saussure's diagram of the sign into the formula <S/s>. I understand Lacan's theory of signifier, its primacy with respect to the signified, as a crucial step forward to his later conceptualization of discourse.

In Sect. 5.2.2, "Enter the Analyst", I highlight the way Lacan's understanding of language shifts from a structure of signifiers to a discursive relation of signifiers that always produce a signifying remainder. For Lacan, the arbitrary relation between signifier and signified is unstable and shifting which illustrates how the apparently fixed relation between a signifying element and a concept constantly slides under the signifier. I emphasize the transformative function of the master signifier in the Analyst's discourse as putting a temporary halt to the metonymic sliding characteristic of the signifying chain. In the Analyst's discourse master signifiers are produced by the subject, rather than being imposed on subjects from the outside. I connect Lacan's notion of the *point de capiton* with the function of the master signifier in the Discourse of the Analyst in that it provides a means to reconfigure the previously closed order of

[2] See also Lacan's essay "The Function and the Field of Speech" (1953).

signifiers and so to reorganize signification around the production of a new signifying chain.

The title "Between Reality and the Real" refers to two interrelated themes. On the one hand, Lacan negates the notion of a pre-discursive reality and presents the reality of the world as being already inscribed in discourse. This means that the speaking subject does not emerge in a neutral space but is inserted rather into existing relations where s/he must contend with the realities of social life. On the other hand, Lacan's concept of discourse provides a trenchant critique of a structural totality and exposes the impossibility of language to completely fix the categories and identities through which subjectivity and social reality are produced. The Analyst's discourse is informed by Lacan's definition of the Real as an impossible plenitude; the master signifier it produces is thus open, fluid, and processual. The psychoanalytic discourse accepts the fact that it cannot fully know or represent the Real while also accepting that it offers a multiplicity of possibilities for language to represent a different relationship to the Real.

5.2.1 From a Theory of the Sign to Discourse Theory

From the 1950s, Lacan begins to assert the significance of language as the key to carrying forward Freud's revolutionary approach to psychic subjectivity. Malcolm Bowie notes that Lacan "spends a long time creating from Saussurean raw materials a linguistics fit for psychoanalysis to espouse" (1991, 62). Lacan's essay "The Agency of the Letter in the Unconscious" (1957) outlines one attempt to cross-fertilize Freud's theory with that of the Saussure. Departing from classical linguistics, Saussure utilized a synchronic analysis to explain how linguistic structures produce meaning. His approach rejected the common-sense belief that language is a "naming process—a list of words, each corresponding, to the thing that it names" (1959, 65). Refuting the notion that words have a natural relation to the object they constitute, Saussure developed his binomial definition of the sign. Defined as a "two-sided psychological entity", the sign brings together the sound-realm and the thought-realm of two logically commensurate notions: the signified (concept), and signifier (acoustic image) (12). In the sign, a signifier and a signified collide and are bonded.

In his 1957 essay, Lacan maps out a new conceptual landscape to give a new rigor to the psychoanalytic account of language while using Saussure as his main theoretical support. Through an inventive reworking of Saussurean concepts, Lacan inverts the algorithm of the sign into the formula <S/s>: "the signifier over the signified, 'over' corresponding to the bar separating the two stages" (*ÉS* 113). For De Saussure, the relationship between the signifier and the signified is initially "arbitrary" and "unmotivated", but once the bonding takes place the sign becomes a fixity, and the two components are thought of as symmetrical and interdependent (1959, 69). Stressing the dissymmetry and disproportion that reign inside the sign, Lacan holds that the signifier is primary and produces the signified. Whence the potency of the signifier which Lacan symbolizes with a single capital "S". Lacan understands the signifier and the signified to correspond to "two distinct orders, separated initially by a barrier resisting signification" (*ÉS* 114). The order of the signifier operates as "a system of differential couplings" which is combined "according to the laws of a closed order" (116).

Commentators point out that Saussure's model is problematic insofar as it appeals to an essential difference between phonic and conceptual substances to explain the formal operations of language (Torfing 1999; Laclau 1994). When viewed independently from one another, the signifier and signified operate at the same level through relations of difference. When viewed together, they produce a positive entity: the sign. The critical theorist Ernesto Laclau argues that asserting an isomorphic relationship between the two registers must "necessarily lead to the collapse of the distinction between the signifier and signified and the dissolution of the category of the sign" (1994, 69). A further consequence of the structural division of the sign into signifier and signified, as Jacques Derrida remarks in *Of Grammatology*, is that it perpetuates the metaphysical distinction between the "sensible and the intelligible" while implicitly privileging the place of the signified as the site of meaning (1982, 13).[3] Lacan's formula

[3] The partitioning of the sign serves the purpose of isolating meaning or "intelligibility" from the merely sensible signifier.

<S/s> attempts to radicalize Saussure's theory of the sign by showing how meaning is produced by signifiers; it springs from the signifier to the signified and not vice versa.

According to Jean-Luc Nancy and Phillipe Lacoue-Labarthe in *The Title of the Letter*, Lacan "introduces a resistance such that the crossing of the bar, the relation of the signifier to the signified, in short, the production of signification itself, will never be self-evident" (1992, 36). The bar separating the two terms highlights both the inaccessibility of language to the ideas it tries to express and the inaccessibility of conscious thought to unconscious thought. Lacan rejects the possibility of a direct or preinscribed relation between the signifier and the signified, claiming instead that the signifier can only be defined in relation to other signifiers of "reciprocal encroachments and increasing inclusions" (*ÉS* 116). Differently put, the signified cannot be taken as an unchanging unit of conceptual meaning bound to a particular signifier. Rather, meaning emerges as the effect of the relations between signifiers and their articulations. The identity of a signified is contingent on the diachronic unfolding of signifiers which own their identities to a system of structural relations among signifying elements. In this way, Lacan develops a view of the process of signification as autonomous or algorithmic (Hendrix 2019).

Taking inspiration from the work of Russian-American linguist Roman Jakobson Lacan draws on the poetic functions of metaphor and metonymy to develop his notion of a "signifying chain" that is language itself. Metonymy is constituted in a horizontal, syntagmatic expansion of signifiers in an endless concatenation.[4] Characteristic of language in its full potential, metonymy also reveals that in speech one cannot actualize all possible signifiers. Lacan designates as metonymy "the first aspect of the actual field the signifier constitutes, so that meaning may assume a place there" (*É* 421). Metaphor is the structure that allows for the emergence of meaning. Defined by Lacan as the substitution of "one word for another" (rather than their combination), metaphor shows that each signifier has a whole set of other signifiers attached to it vertically on the

[4] See Russell Grigg (2008) *Lacan, Language, and Philosophy*, Chapter 11, "Lacan and Jakobson—Metaphor and Metonymy" pp. 151–170.

paradigmatic axis (422). The substituting process that takes place between two signifiers is only possible because there is no fixed or prior meaning, or as Lacan put it: "metaphor is situated at the precise point at which meaning is produced in non-meaning" (423).

Lacan compares the chain of signifying elements at work in the order of the signifier to a set of "links by which a necklace firmly hooks onto a link of another necklace made of links" (*É* 418). This dense interlocking chain of signifiers results in what Lacan calls the "incessant sliding (*glissement*) of the signified under the signifier" where each signification refers to another and another, *ad infinitum* (425). The signifier <S> thus creates a meaning, but it can only do so thanks to its relation to other signifying elements; it needs the complementation of other signifiers that can appear in the place kept open by one. In other words, the meaning of <s> is not signified by the signifier <S>; there is always a gap between <S> and <s>. A detour via other signifiers is needed and even then, <s> will always withdraw and never become fully present. The tendency toward metonymic sliding and metaphoric substitution implies that there is no stable, transcendental signified beyond the chain of signifiers that would finally halt the movement and round off the signifying process. All signification is therefore provisional.

Rather than collapsing the distinction between the signifier and the signified, Lacan maintains the autonomy of the former to describe the linguistic functioning of the unconscious. Lacan dispels the quasi-metaphysical perspective according to which the unconscious is the single most unknowable or untheorizable element of all observable features of human psychology and of the psychoanalytic enterprise as such. For Lacan, the unconscious is governed by the rules of the signifier and is comparable in structure to a language.[5] This especially evident in the equivalence Lacan draws between the poetic functions of metaphor and metonymy and the unconscious processes of condensation and displacement, respectively, which are active in both language and dream composition and reveal the unconscious in conscious discourse. Whereas

[5] For Lacan, the unconscious is structured like "*un langage*" not "*une langue*". Although both terms translate into English as "language", the former (*langage*) refers to logics and structures of syntax and semantics that are not necessarily specific to particular languages such as French or German.

metaphor, as a process of condensation, concerns the production of meaning in a discrete instance, metonymy shows how meaning is always deferred or relocated within a signifying chain through displacement. For example, ellipsis involves the omission of a word in a syntax without altering the signification, introducing a gap into the syntactical structure itself.

Lacan attributes the genesis of the unconscious to a "split" in the speaking subject. In "The Position of the Unconscious" (1960) Lacan maintains that the division of the subject "derives from nothing other than that very same play, the play of signifiers –signifiers, not signs" (*PU* 267). Lacan's emphasis on the signifier stems from the fact that there is no subject independent of language. This is not to suggest that the subject is reducible to language, rather the subject exists in a circular relationship in which language has privilege. The subject must represent itself in language to gain access to the symbolic order, but no representation can ever capture the subject completely. The immersion of the subject in the system of the signifier has crucial implications for Lacan's understanding of the unconscious. When Lacan speaks of the unconscious as "the discourse of the Other" he has in mind a group of postulations including: the unconscious is a network of language and rules, the subject is inhabited by the Other, and psychoanalysis is a variety of speech.[6] The term "discourse" underscores the transindividual nature of language; the fact that speech always implies another subject, an interlocutor.

When applied to the concept of discourse, Lacan's thesis "the unconscious is structured like a language" suggests that the same is true of the social field. According to Lacan's formulation in Seminar XVII (1969–1970), discourse does not merely reflect a set of positive preexisting social relations; it constitutes the objects we encounter in reality and articulates the positions that are available to us as speaking beings. For an object to possess a meaningful identity, it must be given a place in relation to other signifying elements within a discourse. Although elements can enter into manifold structural relationships with discourses,

[6] See Lacan's text "The Subversion of the Subject and the Dialectic of Desire in the Freudian Unconscious" (Lacan 2001, pp. 292–325).

their identities are never completely fixed by them. This is where Lacan's insistence on the primacy of the signifier comes into play; in the absence of the structuring force of a signified acting as a stabilizing center, Lacan's account of discourse maintains the openness of the field of discursivity. The shift in Lacan's understanding of language from a "closed order of signifiers" to a discursive relation of signifiers that produce a signifying remainder, allows for a conception of structure as de-centered and undecided due to the constitutive incompleteness of the symbolic order.

5.2.2 Enter the Analyst

The move from a structuralist theory of the sign to the concept of discourse is sometimes regarded as the opening of structure to the unregulated play of relations between signifying elements that may proliferate infinitely and haphazardly. With his term *point de capiton*, variously translated in English as "quilting point", "anchoring point", and "upholstery button", Lacan accounts for the partial fixation of meaning within a signifying chain. One of the earliest references to the term comes from Lacan's Seminar III: *The Psychoses* (1955–1956). In this seminar, Lacan accounts for the fact that in the normal neurotic subject there are certain fundamental points which allow for provisional signification. For a neurotic subject to be considered normal, a minimal number of anchoring points are necessary and "when they are not established, or when they give way" the result is psychosis (1993, 269). By rethinking the diagnostic categories of neurosis and psychosis through the structuring role of language, Lacan begins to blur the distinction between the normal and the pathological. The neurotic subject could be thought of as normal in neurosis, and the psychotic normal in psychosis.

The *point de capiton* is one element that Lacan employs to frame this perspective. It is also the point in relation to which Lacan asserts that "all concrete analysis of discourse must operate" (*SIII* 267). Later associated with "nodal points" in social discourse theory (Laclau and Mouffe 1985; Žižek 2000), Lacan states that "everything radiates out from and is organized around this signifier, similar to these little lines of force that an upholstery button forms on the surface of a material" (*SIII* 268).

Equivalent in function to master signifiers, nodal points establish discourses by setting boundaries for the free play of signifying elements devoid of any fixed meaning. The *point de capiton* stabilizes a group of floating signifiers by linking them into a consistent series in which they acquire meaning in a particular discursive context.[7] Contrary to the notion of a structural totality, the concept of discourse regulated by nodal points recognizes the inevitability of a surplus of meaning that escapes fixation and structural closure.

Within the structure of language meaning is determined according to the temporality of the signifying chain. In Seminar III, Lacan describes the upholstery button as "the point of convergence that enables everything that happens in a discourse to be situated retroactively and prospectively" (*SIII* 268). The dual temporality of retroaction and anticipation structures the way meaning is assigned to phenomena. For example, when a speaker utters the words "the fact remains…", the listener anticipates the sentence's conclusion, which is the moment s/he can grasp the meaning of the speaker's words. Once the speaker has completed the sentence with "…that many facts are dubious", the quilting point retroactively reconstitutes the chain of signification in a direction that could not be anticipated at its inception.[8] Such sentences express meaning, but that meaning is produced via the retroactive effect of the chain's punctuation.

Stressing the diachronic dimension that metonymy introduces into the signified, Lacan remarks that "the signifier, by its very nature, always anticipates meaning by deploying its dimension in some sense before it" (*É* 419). This suggests that meaning fails to keep pace with the unfolding of the chain of signification; it can run ahead, get left behind, circle back, or be continuously delayed. Just as the signified can, through the process of metonymy, slide interminably, so too can the signifier pull away from meaning at the very point where meaning appears to emerge. The precariousness of the signifier embodies the ambivalence of the subject's immersion in a pre-existing language, constraining in advance the meaning that can be made and multiplying the possibilities for that meaning

[7] The term "floating signifiers" refers to signifiers without signifieds. See: Jeffrey Mehlman, "The 'Floating Signifier': From Lévi-Strauss to Lacan", *Yale French Studies* 48 (1972): 10–37.

[8] This example is discussed in Stephany Swale's book "Perversion: a Lacanian Psychoanalytic Approach to the subject" (2012, p. 23).

to exceed the subject's intentions. While forming the necessary support for the emergence of signification, the signifier also threatens to disconnect the networks of meaning, plunging the subject into psychosis.

In Seminar XVII: *The Other Side of Psychoanalysis* (1969–1970), Lacan designates as "master signifier" the fundamental symbolic element which knits the signifier to the signified, thereby arresting their constant sliding (*SXVII* 219). The Discourse of the Master describes the point at which the subject enters the signifying chain through identification with a symbolic term, the *trait unaire*, which marks the subject as a singular and unified identity.[9] In the Master's discourse, the unary trait is symbolized as <S1>: master signifier. For Lacan, the master signifier marks the point of emergence of the subject's speech since the identification with the "I" of speech, the <S1> symbolizing the Master's "I", constitutes the subject's position of enunciation (62). The Master's discourse inaugurates a subject who is identical to the signifier which names it. For this reason, the Master subject perceives itself as a unified "I" capable of mastering its desires, its unconscious, and its others. Such a subject, as Bruce Fink remarks:

> must show no weakness, in this sense carefully hides the fact that he or she, like everyone else, is a being of language and has succumbed to symbolic castration. (1998, 32)

The Discourse of the Master represses the truth of the division of the speaking subject in language.[10] Due to the procedure of repression, the subject refuses knowledge of its formation in signifying networks. Lacan represents this refusal to know with the arrow in his schema <S1> → <S2>.[11] Given this discursive structure, it is impossible for the subject to know its relation to the signifier. The process of symbolic identification with <S1> establishes a subjective relation between the "I" of the

[9] In developing the notion of the unary trait Lacan draws on Freud's account, in *Group Psychology and the Ego* (1921), of the process of the assimilation of an aspect or characteristic of another, in which the subject identifies with a trait of another subject.

[10] Lacan illustrates this repression by placing the divided subject <$> below the bar in the place of truth in the Master's discourse.

[11] In contrast to this schema, the Hysteric interrogates the master signifier <$> → <S2> and thus questions its place within signifying networks.

speaking subject and the ego which appear to be co-extensive, and which produce a positive content: the conscious self of identity. By confusing the ego with self and the self with subject, the Master's discourse takes up a defensive position against the unconscious. With his homophonic construction, "*je suis m'être de moi-même*", Lacan links the "I" (*je*) and ego (moi) with being (*être*) and mastery (*maître*) to illustrate how the production of identity in the Master's discourse generates a socio-symbolic relation of mastery of the subject to itself and to other subjects (*SXVII* 79).

In the same way that Lacan denies the possibility of fixing the identity of signifying elements in a discourse through reference to a stable, transcendental signified, he also opposes any philosophy in which consciousness founds the illusion of a "transcendental 'I'" (*SXVII* 62). This enunciative position, made readily available by the Master's discourse, is characterized by the imaginary permanence and stability of the ego. For Lacan, the refusal of the unconscious implies that signification does not cross the bar of signification between signifier and signified. By contrast, in the metaphoric substitution of one signifier for another, Lacan explains that "the effect of signification is produced that is creative or poetic [...] which is the advent of the signification" (*ÉS* 125). By resisting the movement of metaphor, the Master's discourse dictates that relations between signifiers remains the same. Deprived of the enunciative position to produce a new signified, the subject can only reproduce the symbolic economy of the Master.

Dethroning the subject of consciousness from its primary position, Lacan's theory of the four discourses foregrounds the "subject of the signifier" which he previously linked to the unconscious (*SXVII* 4). In his text, "The Subversion of the Subject and the Dialectic of Desire" (1960), Lacan describes the unconscious as "a chain of signifiers which [...] is repeated, and insists on interfering in the breaks offered it by the effective discourse and the cogitation that it forms" (*ÉS* 227). For Lacan, the unconscious intervenes in conscious discourse and structures the production of signification. Kirsten Campbell insightfully explains that the "signification of the knower [is] marked by what it cannot represent, because its signification is always in (unconscious) excess of what it consciously intends to represent" (2004, 38). In the Master's Discourse the unconscious speech of the subject, <$>, subtends its conscious speech which, in turn, produces a left-over: <*a*>. In this way, Lacan shows that the term <*a*> represents both the unassimilable excess to discourse and the gap in the symbolic structure.

Dylan Evans states that "no matter how many signifiers one adds to the signifying chain, the chain is always incomplete; it lacks the signifier which could complete it" (1996, 96). In supposing a formalization of discourse in Seminar XVII, Lacan encountered the exclusion of an "element of impossibility" that founds and structures all discourses (*SXVII* 45). In the Master's discourse, the <*a*> stands for the excluded term. The <*a*> functions as the gap in the Symbolic structure whose exclusion by the Discourse of the Master masks the basic fact that it is impossible to "say it all". The Master subject structures its relation to this unassimilable excess by rendering it as an imaginary object (*objet a*): the conscious self of identity. By contrast the unconscious has no such positive content; it marks the void or inconsistency between the symbolic elements of language. Lacan's account of the discursive structure as constitutively incomplete offers the possibility to change the structure of signifiers that produce the subject. Change does not depend on securing or fixing identity but rendering it mobile.

In contrast to the fixity and rigidity of the Master's discourse, Bruce Fink explains that the Discourse of the Analyst "is opposed to all will of mastery, engaging in a continuous flight from meaning and closure in a displacement that never ceases (1995, 124). The Analyst's discourse brings the excluded term, <*a*>, into the dominant position. In psychoanalysis, the analysand is invited to articulate the structure of signifiers that produce it as subject. The re-inscription of the symbolic <*a*> into the analysand's signifying chain permits a reconfiguration of signifiers and a reorganization of signification through the production of a new signifying chain. Lacan represents this new discursive structure with his schema <*a*> → <$>. The Analyst's discourse inverts the lower level of the Master's discourse that contains Lacan's formula for fantasy <$ Δ *a*>. The analyst enables the analysand to traverse the imaginary <*a*> which underpins the analysand's identity and establishes the fixed structure of its discourse.

Analysis involves a process in which the analysand brings into its symbolic system the signifiers of the Other, or as Lacan previously put it: "in order to free the subject's speech, we introduce him into the language of his desire" (*ÉS* 60). Rather than taking a defensive position against the unconscious and desire, the analysand "speaks" them in order to change them. Kirsten Campbell claims that "the articulation of the Other" restores the mobility of the signifying chain because it opens that structure to the richness of metaphoric substitution" which founds the productivity of signification (2004, 41). In this account, the production of meaning is supple, mobile, and mutable, as in the Analyst's discourse. With <S1> as its discursive product, Lacan intends to underscore the possibility of changing the structure of signifiers that produce the subject. If the master signifier is the material through which the subject assigns meaning to the Real; then changing the subject's relation to the signifier also changes the subject's relation to the Real. Through the production of a new signifying chain, the Discourse of the Analyst holds out the possibility of signifying the Real differently. According to Lacan, a new relation to the Real produces a change at the level of the subject's "being":

> The slightest alteration in the relation between man and the signifier [...] changes the whole course of history by modifying the moorings that anchor his being. (*ÉS* 132)

In what follows, I consider the change in the relation between the subject and the signifier in terms of a new discursive structure and so a new subject position.

5.3 A Retroactive Constitution of Meaning

In this section, I address the passage of Foucault's discourse from Hysteric to Analyst. I situate Foucault's position as a discoursing subject within the critical tradition of Kantian philosophy. Within this symbolic economy, "Kant" functions as a kind of master signifier. Reading Foucault's discursive position in relation to the signifier "Kant" introduces us into symbolic knowledge which implies knowledge (*savoir*) of the subject's subjection to the signifier (Campbell 2004). I identify "Kant I" as the signifier to which Foucault, in the Hysteric's discourse, is subjected; it stands for a transcendental legacy, a search for universal values, and the conditions of possibility of true knowledge. I claim that "Kant II" is the signifier which enables Foucault to engage in a practice of symbolization that marks his transition to the Analyst's discourse; it signifies an alternative to the "blackmail of Enlightenment",[12] a "critical ontology of ourselves" in the present,[13] and a point of reference for imagining a philosophy of the future. What gives the nodal point "Kant" its readability is Foucault's discursive positioning. I read "Kant" not as a fixed referentiality, but a signifier in relation to which Foucault constitutes himself as a discoursing subject in the process of change.

In the Analyst's discourse, the analysand as knowing subject is the "barred" subject of the unconscious who critically articulates the existing orders of representation into which s/he is inserted and the cost of entering those symbolic economies. Refusing the comforts of a stable and reassuring identity, the analysand recognizes instead his or her temporality, disunity, and division. In Sect. 5.3.1, "The Kantian Division Revisited", I consider the repeated attempts Foucault makes throughout his career to situate his intellectual work, and the French lineage to which it belongs, in a complex and often contentious relation to Kant's philosophy and the discourses of modernity more generally. This allows me to illustrate the slippage of signification in which the signifier "Kant" has a shifting and contingent signified with no referent. I highlight examples from the late 1970s and early 1980s in which Foucault situates the referent of "Kant" in both a present and future signifying relation to the Real.

In Section 5.3.2, "Tutelage and the Way Out", I apply Lacan's notion of the *point de capiton* to my reading of Foucault. For Lacan, the *point de capiton* marks the point in the signifying chain at which "the signifier stops the otherwise endless movement of signification" and produces the necessary illusion of a fixed meaning (2001, 231). I identify Foucault's

---

[12] In his text "What is Enlightenment", Foucault describes the charges brought against him by his critics in the following way: "you either accept the Enlightenment and remain within the tradition of its rationalism [...] or you criticize Enlightenment and then try to escape from its principles of rationality" (Foucault 1997, pp. 120).

[13] In his lecture course "The Government of Self and Others" (1982–1983), Foucault opposes two Kantian traditions. The first poses the question of the conditions of true knowledge. The second concerns the question of present reality and the field of possible experience. Foucault locates in this second tradition "the ontology of ourselves" which he opposes to the first Kantian tradition, pp. 20–21.

lecture course "The Government of Self and Others" (1982–1983) as site of the chain's punctuation in which the signifier and the signified are knitted together. In his opening lecture, Foucault distinguishes between two Kantian legacies: (1) a transcendental legacy, to which he refuses to subscribe, which establishes universal rules of truth; (2) a historico-critical legacy, in which he situates himself, that challenges the present based on the diagnosis of what we are. I argue that Foucault's self-insertion in the second tradition (Kant II) performs a resignification of the discourses of modernity and effects a restructuration of the past contingent traces of the signifier "Kant" (I) which makes readable his new positioning within the Discourse of the Analyst. Informed by Lacan's theoretical perspective of the four discourses, I insert my reading into a growing body of interpretive literature concerning Foucault's connection with Kant.

I present this discussion under the Sect. 5.3 heading "A Retroactive Constitution of Meaning". Due to the diachronic unfolding of the chain of signifiers, the *point de capiton* foregrounds a retroactive signification whose function Lacan illustrates in the elementary cell of the graph of desire pictured below. The graph illustrates how the vector of pre-symbolic intention <Δ> enters the signifying chain <S—S′> at an ulterior point and leaves it an anterior point with the subject <$> (Zupančič 2000). Applied to Foucault, I understand the temporal movement of the *capitonnage* in terms of the movement of metaphor –the moment when the signifier crosses the bar and knots the signified, revealing the signification of the term "Kant" (Fig. 5.1).

The quilting point appears when a number of signifying elements that were floating around previously are linked together into a consistent series and given a new meaning. The Analyst's discourse is distinguished by the fact that master signifiers are produced by the subject, rather than being imposed on subjects from the outside. I signal the intervention of the *point de capiton*, as marking the passage of Foucault's discourse from that of the Hysteric to that of the Analyst to stress the productive and transformative function of the signifier. To the extent that the Analyst's discourse provides a means to reconfigure the previously closed order of signifiers and so to reorganize signification around the production of a new signifying chain <S1>, I claim that Foucault's resignification of the term "Kant" (II) can be situated there.

Graph I

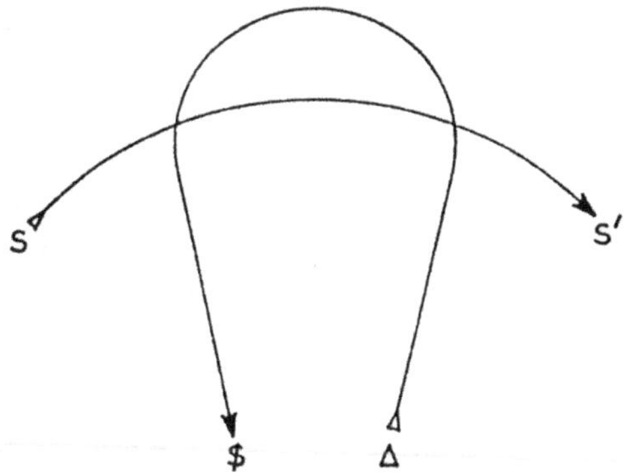

Fig. 5.1 Lacan's basic graph of desire

5.3.1 The Kantian Division Revisited

Foucault's engagement with Kant consists not of a single treatise but of snippets scattered throughout his work, written at diverse lengths and in a variety of contexts. The pieces that appear in Foucault's written publications in the mid–1960s are marked by their explicit criticism of Kant's contribution to Enlightenment philosophy. One example can be found in Foucault's (1966) review of Ernst Cassirer's *Philosophie der Aufklärung which appeared in the Quinzaine littéraire* under the title "Une histoire restée muette".[14] In this article, Foucault praised Cassirer's study of the Enlightenment which grappled with historical rather than epistemological questions that Kant inaugurated, and which have become fundamental to the constitution of modern thought in the West. Whereas Kant asked how science was possible, Cassirer, Foucault claims, asked how this "Kantianism to which we appear to belong was possible" (*DÉ* 549). The implication, as James Schmidt insightfully observes, is the characterization of Cassirer as a "neo-Kantian" which signifies for Foucault:

[14] The article is included in the 2012 digital edition of *Michel Foucault: Dits et* Écrits, I, *1954–1975*, pp. 547–551.

> The inability of Western thought to overcome the break effected by Kant; neo-Kantianism (in this sense, we are all neo-Kantians) is the ever-repeated injunction to reiterate this break—both to recover its necessity and to understand its consequences more fully. (*DÉ* 547)[15]

The privileging of historical rather than epistemological questions can be observed in Foucault's lecture course "The Will to Know" (1970–1971). Against Aristotle's notion of the naturalness of the desire to know—of the natural access to truth –, Foucault presents the Nietzschean conception of the historical specificity and the production of truth. Commentators remark that Foucault's focus on the political and social transformations in ancient Greece encompasses a more general aim to demonstrate that Kantian philosophy is in fact a contingent result of a particular historical set of social changes and political conflicts (Andía 2015). In his 1966 article, Foucault describes "Kantianism" as the medusa of western thought which blinds us to our own modernity because it emerged at a historical juncture marked by a renewed nostalgia for the Greek world and for the certainties of the eighteenth century (*DÉ* 549). By contrast, the memory of Antiquity that Foucault reconstructs in "The Will to Know" is one of violence and exclusion.[16] Whereas Kant introduced a fundamental antinomy in which the discourse of modernity had to choose between being: "Greek or *Aufklärer*, on the side of tragedy or the *Encyclopédie*, on the side of poetry or well-made language", Nietzsche's "monstrosity", insists Foucault, offers a way out of this dilemma by belonging to both camps at once (549).

This is not the first time that Foucault opposes Nietzsche to Kantianism. Another example comes from Foucault's complimentary doctoral thesis *Introduction to Kant's Anthropology* which he submitted, along with the *History of Madness*, to the Sorbonne in 1961.[17] In this text, Foucault considers the relationship between empirical anthropology and critical

[15] Schmidt's blog entry is available at https://persistentenlightenment.com/2013/07/02/foucault-cassirer/. [Accessed 12 June 2019].

[16] To recall from Chap. 1, Foucault identified both the banishing of the Sophist and Sophistic truth as well as the elision, by Aristotle, of the transgressive dimensions of desire and the body from philosophical discourse.

[17] Foucault's translation of Kant's *Anthropology* and a brief 'historical note' was published by Vrin in 1964.

philosophy. Situating Kant's *Anthropology* in relation to the three *Critiques*, Foucault grasps a notion of "man" specific to the development of modern philosophy. In Foucault's view, it is Kant who inaugurated a new phase of anthropological thinking by relegating the critical investigations to the subject of "man". The question "what is man?" gathers all three critical questions (1) "what can I know", (2) "what should I do", and "what can I hope for" under a single frame of reference. Foucault then asks if "an archaeology of the [*Anthropology*] were possible, would it not reveal the genesis of a *homo criticus*, the structure of which would be different from the image of man that went before" (*IKA* 19–20). According to Foucault, the difference is that "man" now understands himself as both subject and object of knowledge:

> What is in question [...] is the development of self-awareness and of the "I am": the subject self-affecting by the movement in which he becomes aware of himself as an object. (*IKA* 19–20)

Whence the notion of "man" as a modern epistemological concept. One consequence of the recentering of the three critical questions is that Kant's *Anthropology* conveys the notion of a transition from an *a priori* knowledge to an *a priori* experience. Beatrice Han explains that this occurs when the *Anthropology* fuses the empirical with the transcendental: "by placing the transcendental subject [...] within the chronology of empirical objects, the *Anthropology* reveals the transcendental determination as somehow pre-existing itself in the past" (2005, 180). Foucault develops this complex perspective in *The Order of Things* (1966) where he identifies the modern mode of "man's" being in the "empirico-transcendental doublet", the "*cogito*-unthought relation", and the "origin's retreat and return" (*OT* 382). The clarity and distinction of *a priori* knowledge is obscured by an *a priori* experience in which the transcendental subject appears already there, unable to account for the conditions of its own emergence. Highlighting this phase in our anthropological thinking, Han explains that objectivity and subjectivity are "destined to exchange roles in an infinite oscillation between the empirical and the transcendental aspects of man, which invalidates the critical project of giving knowledge limits and a secure foundation" (2005, 181). As a result, Foucault states that:

> The anthropological configuration of modern philosophy consists in doubling over dogmatism, in dividing it into two different levels each lending support to and limiting the other: the pre-critical analysis of what man is in his essence becomes the analysis of everything that can, in general, be presented to man's experience. (*OT* 372)

For Foucault, Kant's *Anthropology* imparts the lesson that the empirical nature of anthropological thinking cannot be grounded in itself; it must refer to the *Critique*(s). Diagnosing what he calls our modern "anthropological sleep", Foucault opposes the anthropological philosophies that emerged after Kant which posit a natural access to truth. In the conclusion to his *Introduction*, Foucault remarks that the "Nietzschean enterprise" provides a new model of critique by bringing "that proliferation of the questioning of man to an end" (*IKA* 124). The upshot of Kant's *Anthropology* is that it enabled Foucault to build an *a contrario* method and conceptual apparatus that works against the humanist tradition of a "founding subject" and the philosophy of an "originary experience" (Han 2002). Following Nietzsche, Foucault highlights the hazardous path of the *will to truth* which fully appreciates the contingent and historically contextualized character of all truth-claims. Foucault later clarifies in "What is Enlightenment" that the aim is to switch from a conception of critique as transcendentally grounded, to a conception of practical critique that is historically specific:

> Criticism is no longer going to be practiced in the search for formal structures with universal value, but rather as an historical investigation into the events that have led us to constitute ourselves and to recognize ourselves as subjects of what we are doing, thinking, saying. In this sense the criticism is not transcendental, and its goal is not that of making a metaphysics possible: it is genealogical in its design and archaeological in its method. (2007, 125)

By tracking the temporal constitution of modern subjectivity alongside the emergence of new knowledges in the human sciences, Foucault shows that any foundation can only appear as a historical beginning, not an origin. Unlike Kant who anticipated the possibility of all knowledge by prescribing universal laws in advance, Foucault begins with the spatially and temporally localized character of already constituted forms of knowledge in order to define retrospectively that which rendered them possible. Under the influence of Nietzsche, Foucault reorients Kant's critical project through an archaeological and genealogical examination of the historical *a priori*(s) of possible experience. Multiple formulations of the historical a priori exist in Foucault's work, from the *episteme* which provides "the total set of relations that unite, at a given time, the discursive practices that give rise to epistemological figures"[18] to a *regime of truth* "which defines the rules according to which true and false are separated".[19] In this way, Foucault opens the space for a new form of critical interrogation which James Bernauer puts in comparison with the three questions listed in Kant's *Critiques*:

> Not "What can I know?," but rather, "How have my questions been produced? How has the path of my knowing been determined?" Not "What ought I to do", but rather, "How have I been situated to experience the real? How have exclusions operated in delineating the realm of obligation for me?" Not "What may I hope for?" but rather, "What are the struggles in which I am engaged? How have the parameters for my aspirations been defined?". (1988, 46)

Foucault follows Nietzsche in demonstrating that our habitual modes of thought and action have a historical beginning and bare the traces of conflicting individual *wills to power* of various people, groups and classes in history. Rather than producing a "critique of pure reason" *à la Kant*, Thomas McCarthy argues that Foucault effectuates a "sociohistorical turn" within the very practice of philosophy (1990, 294). Such a turn, as McCarthy explains, emphasizes "the intrinsic *impurity*" of reason, "its

[18] See M. Foucault (2002b) *The Archaeology of Knowledge*, p. 107.

[19] See M. Foucault (1984) "Truth and Power" in P. Rabinow (ed.) *The Foucault Reader*, p. 73.

embeddedness in culture and society, its engagement with power and interest, the historical variability of its categories and criteria, the embodied, sensuous and practically engaged character of its bearers" (243). Foucault adapts Kant's critique to support his sociohistorical conception of how individuals are constituted in relation to a reality of already given practices of a determinate historical terrain (Olssen 2003). Viewed from this angle, Foucault insists that critique is not a matter of saying that things are not right the way they are, it involves pointing out on what assumptions the practices we accept rest:

> Criticism is a matter of flushing out that thought and trying to change it: to show that things are not as self-evident as we believed, to see that what is accepted as self-evident will no longer be accepted as such. Practicing criticism is a matter of making facile gestures difficult. (*PPC* 155)

A further example of the Kantian break can be observed in Foucault's attempts to situate himself within the tradition of French thought. One example comes from Foucault's introduction to Georges Canguilhem's *The Normal and the Pathological* (1991).[20] In this text, Foucault explains that Canguilhem's work in the history of biology articulates the knowledge about living beings or "life" in general and the "formation of concepts" found in it that express such knowledge (1991, 19). For this reason, Foucault claims that Canguilhem brought the history of science down from its lofty position "toward the middle regions where knowledge is much less deductive, much more dependent on external processes [...] where it has remained tied much longer to the marvels of the imagination" (1991, 19). This text is revealing to the extent that, in it, Foucault begins to present his account of the legacy that contemporary French philosophy inherits from Gaston Bachelard, Jean *Cavaillès* and Canguilhem in the history of science who are, in turn, indebted to Kant and the rest of the philosophy of the Enlightenment.

In developing this point of view, Foucault claims that there are two readings in France which receive Edmund Husserl's phenomenology but

[20] The French version of Canguilhem's *On the Normal and the Pathological* exists in different editions, mainly 1943 and 1966, but Foucault's introduction dates from 1978.

interpret it quite differently. One network of thought concerns the work of Jean-Paul Sartre and Maurice Merleau-Ponty in existential phenomenology. The other modality represents the path laid out by the thinkers in the history of science. The line that separates the philosophical discourse of existential phenomenology from that of the history of science is perhaps another way of recasting the Kantian division. At the end of his introduction, Foucault states that it is "to this philosophy of meaning, subject, and experienced thing that Canguilhem has opposed a philosophy of error, concept, and living being" (1991, 24). In contrast to phenomenology which looks to actual experience for "the original meaning of every act of knowledge", Foucault follows Canguilhem in asking: "can we not, or must we not, look for it in the living being himself" and in the concepts of life that structure our environment (21). That individuals live in a conceptual architecture is precisely what enables them to form and reform concepts from an unfixed point of view while moving things around relationally to make them useful. For Foucault, forming concepts is "one way of living in complete mobility"; rather than immobilizing life; it demonstrates, among living beings, an innovation "who inform their environment and are informed by it outward" (21).

Contrasted with Foucault's concerns in "Une histoire restée muette", the process of (re)forming the concepts that structure the environment of living beings points to those ways in which history might actually "speak". Despite having centers of reference in "regional" and well-defined domains in the history of science, Foucault claims that the works of Bachelard and Canguilhem have functioned as "important centers of philosophical elaboration" in that they bring into play the "question of the Enlightenment which is essential to contemporary philosophy" (1991, 11). Crucially, Foucault states that the philosophy of the living being interrogates forms of rationality that construct and "make universal claims while developing in contingency" (12). The research of the historians of science reveal "universal rationality" as being conditioned and therefore presentable as part of history. The relationship between the French tradition in the history of science and the question of the Enlightenment is given a further elucidation in a modified version of Foucault's introduction to Canguilhem's text.

Published in 1985, Foucault's essay "Life: Experience and Science" presents a revised account of what the philosophy of Enlightenment does.[21] In this text, Foucault considers the responses of Kant and Moses Mendelssohn to the question '*was ist Aufklärung*' which Foucault summarizes in terms of "the moment when philosophy found the possibility of establishing itself as the determining figure of an epoch, and when that epoch became the form of philosophy's fulfilment" (1998, 467). In this sense, the *Aufklärung* is the moment when philosophy and the modern period in which it appears determine and define each other. For Foucault, this is the first time that Enlightenment philosophy questions the status, time, and place of rational thought, referring itself thereby to the "present moment" (468). Struggling to make sense of their present reality, Foucault argues that Kant and Mendelssohn reveal the germinal stages of the possibility to historicizing rationality. Foucault situates the Canguilhem cluster in the human sciences as carrying forward Kant's questioning of the present moment.

In the original introduction to Canguilhem's text, Foucault asserts that Mendelssohn and Kant inaugurated a "philosophical journalism" which, at the time, was one of the major forms of the institutional implantation of philosophy (1991, 9). In 1977, alongside a growing interest in Iranian prisoner affairs, Foucault sought to experiment with his own kind of philosophical journalism. In the context of my argument, this is a significant step to which I want to devote attention. Like the nineteenth century philosophers who published their work in the *Berlinische Monatschrift*, Foucault was commissioned by the Italian newspaper, *Corriere della Sera*, to write and edit a regular feature, titled "Michel Foucault Investigates". Foucault's contract coincided with the Iranian Revolution (1978–1979) which became the sole focus of his journalistic work. Foucault described his work as a *reportages d'idées* (ideas report); a particular way of interrogating contemporary reality in which "intellectuals work together with journalists at the point where ideas and events intersect" (1991, 282).[22]

---

[21] This essay originally appeared in the *Revue de metaphysique et de morale* 90:1 (Jan.–Mar. 1985), pp. 5–14.

[22] See Foucault's article "A Revolution of Bare Hands" in Didier Eribon's (1991) *Michel Foucault*.

Foucault's report on ideas sought to introduce the revolution into the European context in a specific manner.

Iranian historian Behrooz Ghamari-Tabrizi (2016) claims that Foucault saw in the revolution an instance of his own anti-teleological philosophy which departs from the standard progressivist schema of Enlightenment. Rather than affirming the internal logic of a universal history, Foucault's reporting on the Iranian uprisings kept the window of possibilities open through a sustained refusal to subject the revolutionary movement to the logic of historical inevitabilities. The ambiguous character of Iran's revolution is reflected by Foucault's *reportage* in terms of both the singularity of events and the contingency of the ideas that informed them. In contrast with journalists who took comfort in predicting with reassuring certainty the outcome of the revolution, Foucault wished to capture the "splendour" of the moment to the extent that it inscribed the indeterminacy of human action. In an article titled "The Mythical Leader of the Iranian Revolt", Foucault reiterates this view in claiming that:

> I cannot write the history of the future, and I am also rather clumsy at foreseeing the past. However, I would like to grasp what is happening right now, because these days nothing is finished, and the dice are still being rolled. (1991, 288)[23]

Foucault's comment is significant for several reasons. First, it sheds light on the historico-critical dimension of philosophy made available by Kant and Mendelssohn. According to Foucault, this entails two objectives that cannot be dissociated from each other. On one hand, it involves locating the moment when the West first asserted "the autonomy and sovereignty of its own rationality" (1991, 10). On the other hand, it requires us "to analyze the present moment" in terms of "what can be its present balance" (10). Through a critical engagement with Enlightenment rationality and the teleological vision of history it envisages, Foucault encouraged his European readers to see the Iranians at the precipice or opening of a transformative politics instead of viewing them as

[23] Cited in Eribon (1991). Foucault's article "The Mythical Leader of the Iranian Revolt" was first published in the *Corriere della Serra*, 26 November 1979.

discursively determined subjects. Second, and related to the first, I claim that Foucault effects a restructuration of the discourses of modernity by situating his knowledge not in relation to different pasts, nor in relation to past and present but in the space between the present to which we historically belong and its outside: a future that is open to construct. It is here, in a new signifying relation to the Real, that Foucault's transition from the Discourse of the Hysteric to that of the Analyst becomes visible.

5.3.2 Tutelage and the Way Out

In this section, I draw on Lacan's concept of the *point de caption* to foreground the moment when Foucault constitutes a group of floating signifiers as a meaningful chain. To this end, I focus my attention to Foucault's lecture course "The Government of Self and Others" (1982–1983) where he posits a new relation between Kant's text on the Enlightenment and his *Critique*(s). I understand Foucault's presentation of the *Critique* in this course as imposing a partial fixation of meaning on his earlier formulation of the relation between Kant's *Anthropology* and critical philosophy in which the emphasis shifts and becomes the status of tutelage and the way out. I regard this as an opportunity to highlight the retroactive constitution of meaning whereby Foucault inserts himself in a particular tradition of Kant's critical legacy. Informed by Lacan's account of discourse, I present this discussion as introducing a new perspective into the interpretive body of literature that studies Foucault's connection with Kant.

Shortly before his death in 1984, Foucault provides an uncharacteristically forthright declaration of his own allegiances that trace his intellectual lineage back to Kant. One example can be observed in Foucault's opening lecture of the "The Government of Self and Others" in which he distinguishes between two Kantian traditions that divide modern philosophy.[24] On one hand, there is a transcendental legacy historically

[24] A more cryptic example can be found in Foucault's entry for the *Dictionnaire des philosophes* which he submitted under the pseudonym "Maurice Florence". In this text, Foucault aligns his work with Kant and defines his *critical history of thought* as an "analysis of the conditions under which certain relations of subject to object are formed or modified, insofar as those relations constitute a possible knowledge [*savoir*]" (1998, 459).

linked to the *Critique* which poses the question of the conditions of possibility of true knowledge. On the other hand, there is a legacy of critical thought, linked to Kant's response to the question of *Aufklärung* and his reflections on the French Revolution, that leads to a "critical ontology of ourselves" in the present (*GSO* 20). Whereas the first tradition involves a formal inquiry into the conditions in which we can have access to truth, the second involves a radical inquiry into the practices we must undertake to transform ourselves to have access to truth. In summary, Foucault states that:

> It seems to me that the philosophical choice confronting us today is the following. We have to opt either for a critical philosophy which appears as an analytical philosophy of truth in general, or for a critical thought which takes the form of an ontology of ourselves, of present reality. It is this latter form of philosophy which, from Hegel to the Frankfurt School, passing through Nietzsche, Max Weber and so on, has founded a form of reflection to which, of course, I link myself insofar as I can. (*GSO* 21)

For some, this claim is rather striking since Foucault was (and, in some circles, still is) viewed as a critic and perhaps an outright enemy of Enlightenment philosophy. James Schmidt and Thomas E. Wartenberg recall that Foucault spent much of his career "showing that every alleged victory of enlightenment marked the triumph of a new and insidious form of domination" (1994, 284). In their attempts to reconcile Foucault's claims to Kantian affiliation, some scholars conclude that he contradicted himself in one or more ways (Habermas, 1987; Fraser, 1989). Other commentators find coherence in Foucault's criticism of Kant's critical philosophy, arguing that rather than constituting a total rejection, Foucault sought to transform some of its aspects from within (Hendricks, 2008; Allen, 2008). These debates spawn a multiplicity of registers for reading and interpreting Foucault's work in connection to Kant, with each establishing a relation of opposition, contradiction, or reconciliation with the other.

For instance, Habermas understands Foucault's late self-affiliation with Kant as evidence of the need for a normative framework that his work nevertheless invalidates. For Habermas, Foucault entangles himself in a contradiction when he opposes the critique of power to the analytic of truth in such a way that "the former is deprived of the normative standard it would have to derive from the latter" (1989, 154). Habermas interprets Foucault's (re)turn to Kant as an implicit appeal to norms grounded in the philosophical discourse of modernity that he criticizes. Like Habermas, Nancy Fraser argues that Foucault's critique of power presupposes the liberal values which it both requires and rejects (1989, 30). Such criticisms, as John Rachjman remarks, depend upon certain definitions of "modernity" which are contextually specific and historically grounded. Unlike Habermas who thinks of modernity as a repository out of which timeless and universal values may be retrieved, Foucault, argues Rajchman, understands modernity as "an event" and "a critical attitude toward history" (1988, 165). Seen from this angle, it is possible to think of Foucault's engagement with Kant and the discourse of modernity as different from the one that Habermas, informed by a German context, had in mind.

Another form of argumentation comes from Beatrice Han in *Foucault's Critical Project* (2002). In this text, Han argues that Foucault's work can be read as a failed attempt to revive the project of transcendental philosophy by searching for the conditions of possibility for experience. For Han, Foucault approaches this problem in a distinctively historical manner via the historical *a priori* which appears in the context of his archaeological work. Interestingly, Han claims that "despite appearances, archaeology is profoundly connected to phenomenology in that it attempts to find a solution to the same problem" through offering a historicized version of the transcendental (2002, 5). Han reads Foucault as a clandestine Heideggerian grappling with the problems that followed from Edmund Husserl's attempts to grant phenomenology objective grounds. In a later text, "Is Early Foucault a Historian?" (2005) Han provides a revised reading of Foucault as a transcendental-phenomenologist historian and advances the view that:

> *The Order of Things* attempts to re-interpret the Kantian critical project by providing what might be called a transcendental history of the condition of possibility of knowledge in the West. (2005, 586)

In his article "Historicity and Transcendentality", Kevin Thompson reads Foucault through a minority tradition in phenomenology which he calls "phenomenology of the concept" (2008, 1). Thompson locates this tradition primarily in the work of Jean Cavaillès, one of Husserl's most influential readers in twentieth century French epistemology of science. Re-reading portions of *The Archaeology of Knowledge* (1969), Thompson highlights what he takes to be a core concern in Foucault's *critical history of thought*, claiming that: "it seeks nothing less than to grasp the simultaneity of historicity and transcendentality" (2008, 2). In a counter-response to the appropriation of Foucault in favor of various strands of philosophical phenomenology, Gary Gutting (2003) and Colin Koopman (2010) advocate for a pragmatist reading in order to assimilate Foucault into the empiricist tradition. In "Historical Critique or Transcendental Critique" Koopman considers the wider ramifications of these debates on "the relationship of Foucault's projects to Kant's critical philosophy" (2010, 100).

Koopman describes Foucault as a practitioner of Kantian critique but rejects the view according to which Foucault is a philosopher engaged in transcendental inquiry. According to Koopman, commentators who take up Foucault's Kantianism through the lens of phenomenology misleadingly re-interpret archaeology and genealogy as forms of transcendental critique. Koopman, on the other hand, proposes to re-read Foucault's historiographical analytics (both archaeology and genealogy) as an inquiry of how historical conditions of possibility, which are neither universal nor necessary, "constrain thought and action in the present" (2010, 115). In place of transcendentality, Koopman presents Foucault's historiography as a critical project insofar as it constitutes an inquiry into the "problematizations" that condition our present. Differently put, critique for Foucault becomes historical rather than transcendental in orientation. From this perspective, Koopman highlights Foucault's interest in "Kantian critique" and the work he undertook to develop the distinction between two conceptions of critique that can be found in Kant's philosophy, one which he endorses, the other he criticizes.

Amy Allen insightfully captures Foucault's double relationship with Kant in arguing that: "far from a rejection of the Kantian project, Foucault's inversion of Kant's notion of transcendental subjectivity constitutes a critique of critique itself, a continuation-through-transformation of that project" (2008, 24). Similarly, Christina Hendricks understands Foucault's engagement with Kant as a form of "immanent critique" which attempts to transform Enlightenment beliefs and values from within (2008, 360). Taking the line of argumentation one step further, Hendricks maintains that Foucault's self-professed Kantianism is a way to encourage change in his intellectual audience, enabling others "to re-think the role of philosophy and the philosopher to the historically conditioned present" (360). The common thread that unites these perspectives is that Foucault's critique of Kantian critique depends upon a distinction between two "Kants" from which Frederic Gros glosses the following meaning:

> In places there remains the opposition between two possible Kantian legacies: a transcendental legacy to which Foucault refused to subscribe, establishing universal rules of truth in order to avoid the misuses of a dominating reason; on the other hand, a "critical" legacy in which he wants to situate himself, challenging the present on the basis of the diagnosis of "what we are". (*GSO* 379)[25]

Before turning to *The Government of Self and Others* (1982–1983) where Foucault provides the clearest elucidation of the two Kantian traditions, it is important to consider a key element of Foucault's criticism of transcendental philosophy. For Foucault, Kant's transcendentalism is underpinned by an anthropological conception of the subject. Whereas Kant's *Critique* describes the subject as an *a priori* condition of all knowledge, Foucault's reading of the *Anthropology* shows that Kant renders this transcendental subject the object of empirical observation, establishing a basis for the science of "man". Inaugurated by Kant as epistemological concept, "man" emerges in the "analytic of finitude" which Foucault identifies with humanism, a condition of possibility of the modern episteme. For Kant, humanism involves the claim that "man" exists at the center of the universe as a finite being who can reason within limits s/he cannot go beyond. Such a notion produces insoluble contradictions for

---

[25] Gros' comments can be found in the "Course Context" of the *Government of Self and Others.*

the human sciences which are based on incompatible definitions of what "man", history, and thought are. Providing a warped and twisted form of reflection, humanism takes the anthropological conception of the subject as the starting point for a natural access to truth.

For Foucault, "man" cannot serve as the foundation or origin or condition of possibility for anchoring objectivity and truth. Foucault opposes Kantian humanism in the same way he opposed the Cartesian conception of an atomized and disembodied *cogito* set apart from history. It is against anthropological humanism that Foucault's criticism of Kantianism finds its concrete expression, and which takes various forms in Marxism, existentialism, phenomenology as well as Nazism and Stalinism. The anthropological sleep that Foucault describes can only be overcome if Kant's notion of transcendental subjectivity is jettisoned, or rather inverted. Such an inversion entails a commitment to philosophical anti-humanism. Rather than insisting on the priority of "man" whose rational capacities are asocial and ahistorical, Foucault's Nietzschean conception of the subject has no essence, no unity or integral identity. The notion that subjectivity can be embodied in a non-identity which poses a riddle ("who am I") to the anthropological conception of "man", establishes a crucial link to Lacan's account of the divided subject in the Hysteric's discourse in Seminar XVII (1969–1970).

Foucault's criticism of Kant's transcendental philosophy and the anthropological humanism which structures it only partially captures his relation to Kantian critique. The story, in other words, does not end there. In the *Government of Self and Others* Foucault distinguishes between two Kantian legacies in a way that compels him to return to Kant's *Critique*, as if putting a punctuation on his earlier engagement. Only this time Foucault does not return to the *Critique* in reference to the *Anthropology* as before, but in the context of Kant's response to the question of *Aufklärung*. Foucault emphasizes the German word that Kant used to define Enlightenment: *Ausgang*. The French equivalent, "*sortie*", is translated in English as "a way out" and variously expressed in terms such as "release" and "exit". *Ausgang*, explains Foucault, is "a movement by which one extricates oneself from something, without saying anything about what one is moving towards" (2010, 27). Inscribed within this movement is the thing which has meaning for the person who speaks as a thinker, and which constitutes the significant element of his/her present reality. This form of philosophical reflection is not anthropological ("*was ist der Mensch*") but historico-critical, a way of defining the present as *der Ausgang des Menschen*.

With *der Ausgang des Menschen* as a new focal point, Foucault returns to the signifying chain concerning "Kant" and establishes a new relation between the *Aufklärung* and the *Critique*(s). According to Foucault, the "critical enterprise and the process of *Aufklärung* complement each other, summon each other, and render each other necessary" (*GSO* 31). In developing this view Foucault foregrounds Kant's response to the question of *Aufklärung*: "man's way out of self-incurred tutelage" (26). Summarizing what it means to be in "the condition of tutelage", Foucault refers to the three *Critiques* in order to grasp Kant's definition: "the inability to make use of [one's] understanding without the direction from another" (26). Differently put, the critical side and the *Aufklärung* side of *Verstand* correspond to each other in the form of complementarity but also, as Foucault claims, "insofar as it is because we go beyond the legitimate limits of reason that we are led to appeal to an authority" (31). These two sides are precisely what "Kant opposes in the *Critique* and from which the process of *Aufklärung* must deliver us" (31). Foucault thus infers that "tutelage and the way out are in substance" (36).

The link between *Aufklärung* (the way out…) and the *Critique* (…of tutelage) has yet to be fully appreciated by the interpretive literature that explores Foucault's connection with Kant. The "Government of Self and Others" is a crucial reference since it also marks the point at which Foucault articulates a distinction between two forms of Kantian critique. In my reading of Foucault, I choose to interpret this moment through Lacan's notion of the *point de capiton* which describes the effect that follows when the vector of subjective intention retroactively quilts or fixes the vector of the signifying chain. In analysis, this happens when the subject recognizes, in a contingent series of signifiers, the meaning of his/her existence (Zupančič 2000). For the Lacanian analyst, interpretation is directed "not so much at the meaning as towards reducing the non-meaning of signifiers" (*SXI* 212). What matters, as Lacan insists, is for the subject to recognize "to what irreducible, traumatic non-meaning he is as a subject subjected" (251). For Foucault, the production of a new signifying chain arguably represents a new relation to the Real, a relation moreover, that retroactively determines the non-meaning of the signifier "Kant I". Foucault's passage of discourse from that of the Hysteric to that of the Analyst refers this non-meaning to an understanding of positioning as a discursive process that situates Foucault's philosophical project and methodologies of critique within a continuum.

References

Allen, A. (2008) *The Politics of Our Selves: Power, Autonomy, and Gender in Contemporary Critical Theory*. New York: Columbia University Press.
Andía, J. R. (2015), *Michel Foucault,* Review *of Foucault's Lectures on the Will to Know*. http://journals.openedition.org/lectures/18113 [Accessed: 20 January 2021].
Bernauer, J., & Rasmussen, D. (1988) *The Final Foucault*. Cambridge: MIT Press.
Bou Ali, N., & Goel, R. (2020) *Lacan contra Foucault: Subjectivity, Sex and Politics*. New York: Sydney Bloomsbury Academic.
Bowie, M. (1991) *Lacan*. Cambridge: Harvard University Press.
Campbell, K. (2004) Jacques Lacan and Feminist Epistemology. London: Routledge.
Canguilhem, G. (1991) *The Normal and the Pathological*. Translated from the French by C. R. Fawcett with R. S. Cohen. New York: Zone Books.
Copjec, J. (1994) *Read My Desire: Lacan Against the Historicists*. London: Verso.
De Saussure, F. (1959) *Course in General Linguistics*. Translated from the French by W. Baskin, Bailly C., & Sechehaye, A. (eds.). New York: Philosophical Library.
Derrida, J. (1982) *Of Grammatology*. Translated from the French by G. Spivak. Baltimore: John Hopkins University Press.
Eribon, D. (1991) *Michel Foucault*. Translated from the French by B. Wing. Cambridge: Harvard University Press.
Evans, D. (1996) *An Introductory Dictionary of Lacanian Psychoanalysis*. New York/London: Routledge.
Fink, B. (1995) *The Lacanian Subject between Language and Jouissance*. New Jersey: Princeton University Press.
Fink, B. (1998) "The Master Signifier and the Four Discourses", in Nobus, D., (ed.) *Key Concepts of Lacanian Psychoanalysis*. London: Rebus.

Foucault, M. (1990) *Politics, Philosophy, Culture Interviews and Other Writings 1977–1984*. Kritzman, L. D. (ed). New York: Routledge.
Foucault, M. (1991) *Remarks on Marx: Conversations with Duccio Trombadori*. Translated from the French by R. J. Goldstein, & J. Cascaito. New York: Semiotext(e).
Foucault, M. (1994a) *The Order of Things: An Archaeology of the Human Sciences*. Translated from the French by A. Sheridan. New York: Vintage Books.
Foucault, M. (1994b) *Dits et écrits, 1954–1969*, vol. 1. Paris: Gallimard.
Foucault, M. (1997) *Ethics: Subjectivity and Truth*, Paul Rabinow (ed.). Translated from the French by R. Hurley and others. New York: New Press.
Foucault, M. (1998) *Aesthetics, Method, and Epistemology* (*Essential Works of Foucault*, 1954–1984, *Vol. 2*), Faubion, J. D. (ed.). Translated from the French by R. Hurley. New York: The New Press.
Foucault, M. (2007) *The Politics of Truth*, Lotringer, S. (ed.). Translated from the French by L. Hochroth & C. Porter. Los Angeles: Semiotext(e).
Foucault, M. (2008) *Introduction to Kant's Anthropology*, Nigro, R. (ed.). Los Angeles: Semiotext(e).
Foucault, M. (2010) *The Government of Self and Others: Lectures at the Collège de France, 1982–1983*, Gros, F. (ed.). Translated from the French by G. Burchell. New York: Palgrave Macmillan.
Fraser, N. (1989) *Unruly Practices: Power, Discourse, and Gender in Contemporary Social Theory*. Minneapolis: University of Minnesota Press.
Ghamari-Tabrizi, B. (2016) *Foucault in Iran: Islamic Revolution after the Enlightenment*. Minneapolis: University of Minnesota Press.
Grigg, R. (2008) *Lacan, Language, and Philosophy*. New York: SUNY Press.
Gutting, G. (2003) "Review of Beatrice Han, Foucault's Critical Project", *Notre Dame Philosophical Reviews*, 5. Available at: https://philpapers.org/rec/GUTROB [Accessed: 20 January 2020].
Habermas, J. (1987) *The Philosophical Discourse of Modernity: Twelve Lectures*. Translated from the German by F. G. Lawrence. Cambridge: The MIT Press.
Habermas, J. (1989) "Taking Aim at the Heart of the Present: On Foucault's Lecture on Kant's What is Enlightenment?", in J. Habermas, *The New Conservatism: Cultural Criticism and the Historical Debate*, Edited & Translated from the German by S. W. Nicholsen. Cambridge: The MIT Press.
Han, B. (2002) *Foucault's Critical Project: Between the Transcendental and the Historical*. Stanford: Stanford University Press.
Han, B. (2005) *The Analytic of Finitude and the History of Subjectivity*. Translated from the German by E. Pile, *The Cambridge Companion to Foucault*. Cambridge: Cambridge University Press, pp. 176–209.

Hendricks, C. (2008) "Foucault's Kantian Critique: Philosophy and the Present", *Philosophy and Social Criticism,* 34, pp. 357–382.

Hendrix, J. S. (2019) "Jacques Lacan and Language", *Architecture, Art, and Historic Preservation,* Faculty Publications, 44.

Koopman, C. (*2010*) "Historical Critique or Transcendental Critique in Foucault: Two Kantian Lineages", *Foucault Studies,* 8, pp. 100–121.

Lacan, J. (1978) *The Seminar of Jacques Lacan, Book XI: The Four Fundamental Concepts of Psychoanalysis,* J. A. Miller (ed.). Translated from the French by A. Sheridan. New York/London: W. W. Norton & Company.

Lacan, J. (1992) *The Seminar of Jacques Lacan,* Book VII: The Ethics of Psychoanalysis, J. A. Miller (ed.). Translated from the French by D. Porter. New York/London: W.W. Norton & Company.

Lacan, J. (1993) *The Seminar of Jacques Lacan, Book III: The Psychoses, 1955–1956,* J. A. Miller (ed.). Translated from the French by R. Grigg. New York/London: W. W. Norton & Company.

Lacan, J. (1995) "The Position of the Unconscious", in R. Feldstein, B. Fink, & M. Jaanus (eds.) *Reading Seminar XI: Lacan's Four Fundamental Concepts of Psychoanalysis.* Translated from the French by B. Fink. Albany: SUNY Press, pp. 259–277.

Lacan, J. (2001) *Écrits: A Selection.* Translated from the French by A. Sheridan. London: Routledge.

Lacan, J. (2002) *Écrits.* Translated from the French by B. Fink, in collaboration with H. Fink & R. Grigg. New York: W.W. Norton.

Lacan, J. (2007) *The Seminar of Jacques Lacan, Book XVII: The Other Side of Psychoanalysis, 1969–1970,* Miller, J. A. (ed.). Translated from the French by R. Grigg. New York: W.W. Norton and Company.

Laclau, E., & Mouffe, C. (1985) *Hegemony and Socialist Strategy: Towards a Radical Democratic Politics.* London: Verso.

Laclau, E., & Zac, L. (1994). "Minding the Gap: The Subject of Politics", in Laclau, E. (ed.) *The Making of Political Identities.* London/New York: Verso, pp. 11–39.

McCarthy, T. (1990). "The Critique of Impure Reason: Foucault and the Frankfurt School", *Political Theory,* 18 (3), pp. 437–69. Available at: http://www.jstor.org/stable/191596. [Accessed: 12 February 2020].

Olssen, M. (2003) "Foucault and Critique: Kant, Humanism and the Human Sciences", in Peters, M. A., Olssen, M., & Lankshear, C. (eds.) *Futures of Critical Theory.* New York: Rowman & Littlefield, pp. 73–102.

Rajchman, J. (1988) "Habermas's Complaint", *New German Critique,* 45, pp. 163–191.

Schmidt, J., & Wartenberg, T. E. (1994) "Foucault's Enlightenment: Critique, Revolution, and the Fashioning of the Self", in Kelly, M. (ed.) *Critique and Power: Recasting the Foucault/Habermas Debate*. Cambridge: MIT Press.

Swales, S. (2012) *Perversion: A Lacanian Psychoanalytic Approach to the Subject*. New York: Routledge.

Thompson, K. (2008) "Historicity and Transcendentality: Foucault, Cavaillès, and the Phenomenology of the Concept", *History and Theory*, 47 (1), pp. 1–18.

Torfing, J. (1999) *New Theories of Discourse: Laclau, Mouffe, and Zizek*. Oxford: Blackwell Publishers.

Žižek, S. (2000) "Class Struggle or Postmodernism? Yes, please!", in Butler, J., Laclau, E., & Žižek, S. (eds.) *Contingency, Hegemony, Universality*. London: Verso, pp. 90–135.

Zupančič, A.(2000) *The Ethics of the Real: Kant and Lacan*. London/New York: Verso.

6

The Parrhesiastic (P)act

6.1 Introduction

When Lacan introduces his Seminar XV: *The Psychoanalytic Act* (1967–1968), he claims to be introducing something new into the analytic discourse concerning the elective moment when an analysand effects the move to psychoanalyst. From the outset Lacan insists that an "act" differs from an action in that it radically transforms the agent; the subject in analysis does not return to the position of analysand once s/he has "acted". In this chapter, I develop the perspective that psychoanalysis, as a praxis, is an act that transpires inside the frame of speech which depends on the position of the Analyst to maintain that frame. To this end, I chart the consideration, on the part of both Lacan and Foucault, of an ethics of speaking or an ethics of the discursive act. I distinguish this act from an ethics of coincidence with oneself or one of confession and self-disclosure through reference to Foucault's analysis of the Greek and Hellenistic concept of *parrhesia* in "The Government of Self and Others" (1982–1983). Drawing a parallel with Lacan, I argue that Foucault develops an ethics

J. L. Davis, *Reading Foucault Through Lacan*, The Palgrave Lacan Series,
https://doi.org/10.1007/978-3-031-69738-8_6

in which speech introduces a disruption, a critical interruption, a dissonance which modifies the mode of being of the subject.

Chapter 6 begins by raising the distinctly modern dimension of ethics in relation to which Lacan and Foucault inscribe the "ethico-political" stakes of their work. Prior to his discussion on the psychoanalytic act, Lacan devotes an entire seminar to "The Ethics of Psychoanalysis" (1959–1960) where he formulates his own analytic ethic that relates desire to action. In this seminar, Lacan presents psychoanalysis as an ethical theory of what is beyond the pleasure principle. In traditional ethics, pleasure principles are central to discussions on the proper measure of pleasure in the notion of the good life and the debates on how to harmonize our interests with the world and each other. For Lacan, we cannot formulate such a principle for our desire because desire will always satisfy itself in ways we cannot regulate. In Sect. 6.2.2, "The Duplicity of Pleasure as Pain", I identify the polymorphously perverse origins of desire as playing a crucial role in Lacan's account of the ethics of psychoanalysis in that it frees us from the domination of pleasure principles that order our lives and tell us how to live.

Foucault's entry into ethics develops out of a crucial shift in his analysis of power relations during his courses at the Collège de France in the late 1970s. Through a major recasting and consolidation of his core conceptual tools, Foucault starts to distinguish "strategic games of power" from "static states of domination" and inserts between these two "the technologies of government" (1997, 283). Foucault employs the term "governmentality" to emphasize the freedom of the subject and its relationship to others which constitutes the domain of ethics. Like Lacan, Foucault argues that there can be no moral system in modernity based on firm foundations concerning the nature of human beings and, thereby, a basis for human action. Foregoing a transcendent ground for ethics, Foucault defines freedom or *liberté* as the ontological condition of ethics; an opening for change that makes possible normalizing modes of existence as well as transformative ones. In Sect. 6.2.1, "Why it Matters that Everything is Dangerous", I stress the mutability of power relations that underpin the exercise of freedom and the dangers inherent in the practices in which we engage to resist oppressive structures.

I present this discussion under the Sect. 6.2 heading "On Modern Ethical Problems" to underscore the absence of any foundation or transcendent ground on which to base contemporary ethics. I identify "freedom" and "polymorphous perversion" as that which determines the ontological precarity—the shifting and uncertain context—in which ethics is called for in the work of both thinkers. For Lacan, psychoanalysis introduces an ethic of what in our sexuality or desire lies beyond the principles that bind us together in the name of a common good or in the form of a common identification. For Foucault, the conditions of freedom, mobility, and mutability that make ethical relations possible uproot myths about the stability and organic unity of a "true self" through the enactment of multiple styles of living. I summarize these points as attempts, made on the part of Foucault and Lacan, to formulate an account of ethics which does not suppose the fixity or rigidity of identity as its ground.

In Sect. 6.3, "The Event of Speech", I highlight the shift, in Lacan and Foucault, from an ethics developed around how to act, to one focused on how to speak. I describe the ethics of speaking as involving a specific form of relation between the speaker and themselves. In Lacan's thought, this relation can be observed in the two positions that the speaking subject occupies in language. That speaking can reveal the difference between the subject of the statement and that of the enunciation implies the division or "split" that is constitutive of the ethical subject for Lacan. In his analysis of ancient *parrhesia*, Foucault understands the two positions in language to establish the basis for an ethical contract of the speaking subject with him or herself in the act of truth-telling. In *parrhesia*, the statement and the enunciation demonstrate that the person who has asserted the truth constitutes themselves as the person who tells the truth through an act that binds him or her to the fact of saying it. I understand the ethics of speaking to produce "retroactive effects" on the speaker who modifies, affirms, or otherwise clarifies his or her mode of speaking insofar as s/he speaks, revealing the difference, in this sense, between the subject who says something and the subjective figure that arises from it.

Starting with Lacan, I evoke the contrast he draws between "full" and "empty" speech to foreground the imaginary and symbolic dimensions of language. I illustrate these concepts through reference to Lacan's diagram of the L-Schema which he introduces in Seminar II: *The Ego in Freud's Theory and the Technique of Psychoanalysis* (1954–1955). I explain how the L-Schema allows us to grasp Lacan's understanding of the act and the relations involved in it between the subject, the other, and the Big Other. I link "full speech" with the aim of psychoanalytic treatment as holding out the possibility for symbolic mediation in order to show how an act can only take on its meaning and status in relation to an encounter of this sort. I provide an example of what "full speech" might mean in the context of Lacan's later account of the *éthique du bien-dire* which he discusses in *Television* (1973). In Sect. 6.3.1, "The Function of the 'I' in the *éthique du bien-dire*", I present this new ethic as one that is correlated with the implication of the speaking subject in the truth that his or her symptom denounces.

The final Sect. 6.3.2, "The Risks of Truth-Telling", asserts the view that Foucault's engagement with *parrhesia* reveals an act of speech which has the function of enacting the speaker's relationship to truth and the reflexivity which the speaker demonstrates towards their own position of enunciation. Rather than defining the "truth" of *parrhesiastic* speech, I stress the emphasis Foucault places on the unspecified risks and dissonance that *parrhesia* opens for the truth-teller. I explain by way of example that *parrhesia* announces those truths which radically destabilize the present by transforming the way being itself is interpreted. The truth in question does not seek to represent a political or social state of affairs, rather *parrhesia* constitutes an "irruptive event" within discourse which allows for transformative sayings without themselves stating the *whole* truth. In this way, I connect Foucault's analysis of *parrhesia*, which foregrounds the status of freedom and the courage of the speaker, with Lacan's assertion in *Television* that truth is related to the Real by what is impossible to say.

Due to the variety of contexts it surveys, this chapter sheds light on the significance of Kant in the work of each thinker. In Lacan's interrogation of the domain of ethics, Kant appears as one of his most important philosophical reference points. On one hand, Lacan admires Kant for establishing a break with traditional ethics by removing morality from the principles that order our lives. On the other hand, Lacan criticizes Kant for turning the moral law into an instrument of the will (or superego). For Foucault, Kant makes possible a different kind of critical philosophy which concerns the conditions and undefined possibilities of the subject's transformation. In the "Government of Self and Others" Foucault positions Kant's text on *Aufklärung* as a sort of prolegomena to the study of the ancient ethical practice of *parrhesia*. In this way, Foucault introduces a specific model of truth-telling that transforms the *ethos* of its interlocutor, carries certain risks for the speaker, and belongs to a temporality of present reality.

6.2 On Modern Ethical Problems

In this section, I consider the distinctly modern dimension of ethics in which Lacan and Foucault inscribe the "etho-political" stakes of their work. Beginning with Foucault, I show how modern relations of power are underpinned by freedom which he takes to be the ontological condition of ethics. Through reference to the concept of "problematization" I discuss how Foucault understands this form of thinking to be an exercise in freedom which becomes the undertaking of ethical practice. I distinguish this exercise from the modern project of rule and modes of self-governing in which the subject experiences his or her own freedom as subjection. I emphasize the precarity or danger of freedom in strategic games of power in order to define the context in which ethics is called for according to Foucault's formulation.

Shifting the focus to Lacan, I consider the status of his thought in the 1960s during which Lacan develops his own analytic ethic that relates desire to action. With Seminar VII: *The Ethics of Psychoanalysis* (1959–1960) as a reference point, I discuss Lacan's insistence that desire has no firm ontological ground. Characterized by its polymorphous perversion, I show how desire is defined by its radical openness rather than any definition of what it opens to. In this way, I explain that Lacan positions psychoanalysis as an ethical theory of what lies beyond traditional pleasure principles. Through his engagement with Kant, I examine the shift in Lacan's thinking from desire to drive in which he links the end of analysis to the concept of the drive, opening thereby a new dimension of psychoanalytic ethics and ethical transformation in the subject.

6.2.1 Why It Matters that Everything Is Dangerous

In an interview conducted by Paul Rabinow and Hubert Dreyfus at Berkeley in April 1983, Foucault was asked whether the ancient Greeks provided a plausible alternative for founding an ethics outside the scientific knowledge about the self, desire, and the unconscious. To this Foucault responds with a definite "no!". In an overview of his work in progress, Foucault explains that the motivation driving his genealogy of ethics is not aligned with the search for alternatives: "I do not want to write the history of solutions" (*EST* 256). It is a question, rather, of doing a "genealogy of problems" which, in Foucault's view, reveals that "everything is dangerous" (256). That danger is always present, describes the context in which ethics is called for: "if everything is dangerous, then we always have something to do" (256). For Foucault, the work of problems or problematizations confronts us with an ethical-political choice which involves determining, on a regular and consistent basis, the main danger that we face today.

The history of problems can be further distinguished from the history of ideas and that of mentalities or behaviors. In a discussion of "Polemics, Politics, and Problematizations" Foucault summarizes the role of thought in the work of problematics with the following statement: "thought is freedom in relation to what one does, the movement by which one detaches oneself from it, constitutes it as an object, and reflects on it as a problem" (*EST* 117). Foucault identifies problematization as constitutive of the activity of a historical ontology of ourselves in the present. A similar formulation is found in *The History of Sexuality, Vol II* (1984) where Foucault explains that human beings "problematize what they are, what they do, and the world in which they live" by taking something (e.g., sexual desire) as an object of concern (*HS2* 10). Crucially, Foucault understands the form of thinking specific to problematization as an exercise of freedom which becomes the undertaking of ethical practice.

Prior to his return to Greek antiquity in the 1980s, Foucault's concern for ethics as an object of genealogical analysis can be linked to a major shift in his understanding of power relations. Between 1976 and 1980, Foucault strengthens his view of power by distinguishing, more precisely, between the strategic conception of power and the states of domination. The Nietzschean conception of forces was a precursor to Foucault's characterization of strategic relations as a play of mobile, reversible, and unstable power. The new modality on which Foucault draws to express the exercise of power at the interior of relationships describes the capacity to structure the field of action of the other and to intervene in the domain of the other's possible action. Maurizio Lazarrato explains that Foucault's account of action upon action "shows what was implicit in the model of battle and war, but that still had not been coherently explained [...]: the virtual freedom of the forces engaged to understand the exercise of power" (2002, 107). In discussion of "The Ethics of the Concern for Self as a Practice of Freedom" Foucault reflects on this period of his work and claims that:

> It seems to me that we must distinguish between power relations understood as strategic games between liberties—in which some try to control the conduct of others, who in turn try to avoid allowing their conduct to be controlled or try to control the conduct of the others and the states of domination that people ordinarily call "power." And between the two, between games of power and states of domination, you have technologies of government—understood, of course, in a very broad sense that includes not only the way institutions are governed but also the way one governs one's wife and children. (*EST* 299)

From this perspective, Foucault understands the power relationship on the basis of two indispensable elements: (1) the recognition of the "other" as a subject who acts, and (2) the field of responses, reactions, effects and possible interventions that may open up as a result. The implication, which Foucault elaborates in "The Subject and Power", is that power is "exercised only over free subjects, and only insofar as they are free" (*SP* 790). Rather than being "trapped" inside of a power relationship, Foucault emphasizes the strategic situation in which free subjects find themselves: "there is always the possibility of changing" (*EST* 167). As indicated in the quote above, the opening and closing of "strategic games" is made possible by the centrality of "governmental technologies" in power relations. Through the exercise of the technologies of government, strategic relations become either static states of domination that are fixed in asymmetric institutionalized relations, or they engender the creation of subjectivities that escape biopolitical power through fluid relations (Lazzarato 2002).

From 1976 to 1979, Foucault delivers a series of lectures at the Collège de France in which he coins the term "governmentality" to designate the operation of power relations that produce incentive structures to conduct the conduct of individuals and populations. In "The Birth of Biopolitics" (1979–1979) Foucault shows that the activity of conducting oneself and allowing one's conduct to be conducted exists in a complex and tangled relationship with economic processes. Governance works not through decrees or injunctions but by establishing areas of convergence between the interests of the state and the interest of individuals. Jason Read remarks that the state "channels flows of interest and desire by making desirable activities inexpensive and undesirable activities costly, counting on the fact that subjects would calculate their interests" (2009, 29). This is especially evident in Foucault's discussions of neoliberal rationality which he analyzes in reference to Gary Becker's theory of human capital. In this theory, Becker describes the government as an enterprise with its central task being to universalize competition and invent market-like systems for the actions of individuals, groups, and institutions. For Foucault the distinguishing feature of neoliberal rationality is "the inversion of the relationships of the social to the economic", which he rhetorically explains:

> What is the function of this generalization of the "enterprise" form? … [I]t involves extending the economic model of supply and demand and of investment-costs-profit so as to make it a model of social relations and of existence itself, a form of relationship of the individual to himself, time, those around him, the group, and the family. (2010b, 242)

One upshot of the term "governmentality" is that it enables Foucault to locate "a relationship of the self to itself, […] and covers the range of practices that constitute, define, organize and instrumentalize the strategies which individuals in their freedom can use in dealing with each other" (1997, 300). The example of subjects governed by neoliberal rationality highlights a freedom that is conditioned by mechanisms of economic interests and the government's skill in managing that freedom. Freedom, in other words, is intrinsic to the modern project of rule which takes the subject as a partner and correlate instrument in its operations (Foucault 2008). This partnership is reflected in the model of economic subjectivity proposed by the Chicago School economists. Foucault describes the shift of *homo economicus* from a partner of exchange (liberalism) to one adapted to entrepreneurial competition (neoliberalism). If the subject is a form made up of a set of characteristics that the individual, in constituting oneself as subject, must recognize as one's own, then Foucault's description of *homo economicus* reflects the ideal form of the neoliberal subject as "an entrepreneur of oneself" (2010b, 226).

For Foucault, governmentality makes it possible "to bring out the freedom of the subject and its relationship to others which constitutes the very stuff of ethics" (1997, 300). Paul Rabinow suggests that it is beginning from this premise that Foucault "understands thought as the exercise of freedom" (*EST* xvii). When applied to Foucault's definition of problematization we can see that neoliberal rationality disavows such an exercise. Governmentality operates most effectively when subjects recognize its regime of truth as their own, and when this truth is experienced as a practice of freedom. The project of rule under neoliberalism is arguably underpinned by an anthropological conception of human beings who have subjectivized the truth that "the market is human nature".[1] To the extent that it is taken as a self-interested decision-making agent imbued with rational calculation, *homo economicus* is presented to us as a natural fact of human existence rather than a contingent effect of power relations that emerged in a particular historical epoch and social circumstances. Even though neoliberal subjects demonstrate the capacity for creativity, flexibility, and openness to change, their self-relation and relationship with others is limited to the economic model of the free enterprise.

The notion that Foucault's foray into biopolitics in the 1970s can be read as a nascent turn towards an *ethos* can be traced back to Deleuze and

---

[1] I borrow this phrase from Fredric Jameson's *Postmodernism; or, the Cultural Logic of Late Capitalism*, p. 263.

Guattari's *Anti-Oedipus: Capitalism and Schizophrenia* (1972). In his introduction, Foucault qualifies this book as a work of ethics and assigns it an alternate title: "An Introduction to the Non-Fascist Life" (1983, xiii). *Anti-Oedipus*, Foucault tells us, is not limited to a particular readership; it is the fact of being anti-oedipal that constitutes a particular *ethos*, a way of thinking and living free from a set of necessary rules that guide our existence. Through reference to an *ethos*, Foucault stresses the creativity and mobility underlying ethical relations and activities. By opposing the *ethos* of *Anti-Oedipus* to fascist ideology, Foucault appears to suggest that ethico-aesthetic practices of self-creation are necessarily critical ones. Indeed, without a critical perspective, we risk tumbling into what Deleuze called "micro-fascism" which Foucault describes as:

> the fascism in us all, in our heads and in our everyday behavior, the fascism that causes us to love power, to desire the very thing that dominates and exploits us. (1983, xiii)

In his genealogy of ethics, Foucault defines the subject not as a substance but a form and insists that "this form is not, above all, or always identical to itself" (*EST* 290). The substance at work in his analysis of ethics are the forms of identity to which subjects are tied both by our own doing and by the institutions, practices, and values of the societies we live in. Fascistic inclinations depend on instances of solidification such as the tendency to consolidate one's identity around points of certainty that provide the foundation for the belief in a "true self". Foucault's ethics proceeds in the opposite direction; it uproots myths about the stability and organic unity of the self. If ethics is to be "the considered form that freedom takes when it is informed reflection", as Foucault defines it, then it must seek to comprehend and counteract the risks, lapses, and potentially destructive tendencies inherent in an *ethos* of opened-ended creation dangers we face in open-ended creation (*EST* 284). Foucault's orientation towards ethics stresses the necessity of rejecting the socially dominant forms of individuality imposed on subjects in order to cultivate a relationship to the self aimed at continual transformation.

Through reference to Foucault's personal life Paul Rabinow claims that he "hopes to invent a mode of subjectivation in which [an] ethos would be a practice of thought formed in direct contact with social and political realities" (*EST* xxxii). The question of sexual orientation provides a further view on this issue. Through his engagement with homosexual practices Foucault's interest in taking the pleasure of sexual relations "away from the area of sexual norms and its categories" holds out the prospect of forming a new culture that escapes "the ready-made formulas of the pure sexual encounter" (*EST* 160). In discussion of "Sex, Power and Politics of Identity" Foucault describes the subculture of sadism and masochism in terms of the innovation it carries for opposing the conflation of sex and pleasure. As a creative endeavor, Foucault understands what he calls the "de-sexualization of pleasure" to be a key feature of S&M in that its practices undermine the conventional idea that "bodily pleasure should come only from sexual pleasure as the root of all possible pleasure" (*EST* 165).

In response to the formation of identities around new sexual practices and their potentially limiting dimension with respect to individuals, Foucault asserts an important distinction. To the extent that "identity" is a procedure to have social and sexual relations that create new friendships, Foucault maintains that it can be useful. If, on the other hand, one's identity becomes the entire problem of social existence, establishing a code and principle to which one must conform, then it falls backs into traditional forms of heterosexual ethics. While it is possible to derive pleasure from identity, Foucault warns against treating identity as "an ethical universal rule" (166). For Foucault, the creation of culture and a new homosexual way of life depends on inventing "the instruments for polymorphic, varied, and individually modulated relationships" that hold out the prospect to "reopen affective and relational virtualities" (*EST* 138). The work of augmenting the freedom, mobility and mutability of these relations takes place within the strategic frame of power. In other words, ethical action involves the interplay of strategic relations in which individuals learn to play the games of power with as little domination as possible in order to maintain (rather than obscure or obstruct) constant recourse to a field of possibilities in which diverse comportments and ways of behaving may be realized.

Games of power, as Foucault understood them, are not intrinsically bad, wrong, or evil. Speaking about his own experience with sexual and amorous relationships, he states: "to wield power over the other in an open-ended strategic game where the situation might be reversed is [...] part of love, passion, and sexual pleasure" (*EST* 298). Through the notion of problematization, Foucault stresses the obligation to reflect critically on the historical forms that make us who we are, and the patient labor required to reformulate them, piece by piece. Such is the work that expresses both the necessity and pleasure of thought. Outside his intellectual life, however, Foucault had difficulty experiencing pleasure and admitted that he struggled to feel it completely. In an interview with Stephan Riggins, Foucault explains that for him *real* pleasure would be something "so deep, so intense, and so overwhelming" that he would not be able to survive it. Foucault recounts an experience which he found pleasurable:

> Once I was struck by a car in the street. I was walking. And for maybe two seconds I had the impression that I was dying and it was really a very, very intense pleasure. The weather was wonderful. It was seven o'clock during the summer. The sun was descending. The sky was very wonderful and blue and so on. It was, it still is now, one of my best memories. (*EST* 129)

Foucault's comments on the pain-inducing aspects of pleasure provide a useful segue into the next section on Lacan.

6.2.2 The Duplicity of Pleasure (as Pain)

In Seminar VII: *The Ethics of Psychoanalysis* (1959–1960), Lacan casts light on the paradoxical origins of desire evinced by the Freudian experience and calls into question the general tendency among analysts to reduce the "polymorphously perverse character of its infantile forms" (*SVII* 4). If the task of psychoanalytic thought is to demonstrate the eventual convergence of these forms in a harmonious conclusion, Lacan asks whether it would not contribute to a new universal moralism focused on the taming of a perverse enjoyment. Stressing the intuition behind Freud's inquiry into the pleasure principle, Lacan positions psychoanalysis as an ethical theory of what lies beyond it; a beyond, moreover, which reveals that human desire has no firm ontological ground. Characterized by its polymorphous perversion, desire is defined by its radical openness rather than any definition of what it opens to (e.g., notions of the good). To the extent that pleasure principles allow us to center our lives in relation to what we think is good, Lacan instructs his analysts to adopt the opposite tendency. Rather than giving patients the "good" they desire, analysts can only give *desire* as such:

> To have carried an analysis through to its end is no more nor less than to have encountered that limit in which the problematic of desire is raised. (*SVII* 300)

Lacan thus formulates his own analytic ethic which relates desire to action, and which he summarizes in the question: "have you acted in conformity with the desire in you?" (*SVII* 314). In Lacan's view, the question of desire can only be posed in the analytic context and "opposed to the pole of desire is traditional ethics" (314). Contrasting his own ethic with traditional moral philosophy, Lacan devotes explicit attention to a line of demarcation introduced by Kant. Prior to Kant, the domain of ethics was problematized at the level of possibility thought in terms of moral obligations which are possible to fulfil. Lacan admires Kant for establishing a markedly different approach to ethics by identifying in morality a demand for the impossible: "an impossibility in which we recognize the topology of our desire" (315). For Lacan, the end of analysis describes the point at which the patient coincides with a libidinal orientation towards an unreachable end. This occurs once the analysand has transformed his or her demand into an acknowledged desire which implies a certain action.

According to Lacan, Kant opened the field of desire onto the realm of the impossible and did so in a way that broke with tradition. Traditional ethics, from Aristotle to Jeremy Bentham, put desires on hold by subjecting the moral subject to a principle of pleasure or happiness. For Lacan, the *Critique of Practical Reason* marks a historical turning point. In his 1963 essay "Kant with Sade" Lacan praises Kant's "radical rejection of the pathological, of any regard for a good, a passion, even a compassion [...] through which Kant liberated the moral law" (*KS* 654). After Kant, the basis of morals is no longer to be sought in the knowledge of pleasure, the good, or the nature of happiness. John Rajchman observes that with Kant morality becomes a matter of "an internal and categorical demand made equally and without exception on each subject, of which it is the task of philosophy to demonstrate the rational foundation or justification" (1986, 49). If psychoanalysis refers to something in our lives which cannot be made into a pleasure principle, then Lacan shows how Kant paved the way for Freud by removing morality from those principles that structured traditional ethical theories and debates.

Lacan argues in Seminar VII that, bound up with the "service of goods", traditional ethics follows a "middle path" which entails "modesty", "temperateness" and "the cleaning up of desire" (1992, 314). Seeking to demystify the Platonic and Aristotelian view of the Supreme good, Lacan provides an account of the historical progression of thought and asserts a direct link between "the domain of the good" and the "economy of goods" (216). Marc de Kesel insightfully points out that when Lacan speaks about the "function of the good" he has "the entire *symbolic* world in mind as both the material and spiritual 'values' and the 'goods' to which we are libidinally bound" (2009, 198). These "goods" respond primarily to our desires and pleasures. In this way, the domain of the good answers to the desire we "are" which Lacan defines as "the desire of the Other". This means that in order for the libidinal being to become a subject s/he must assume the desire of the Other, including all of the goods that the Other desires. Lacan describes how the realm of the good captures the position of desiring subjects:

> The domain of the good is the birth of power. The notion of control of the good is essential [...] To exercise control over one's goods, as everyone knows, entails a certain disorder, that reveals its true nature, i.e., to exercise control over one's goods is to have the right to deprive others of them. [...] For the function of the good engenders, of course, a dialectic. I mean that the power to deprive others is a very solid link form which will emerge the [specific dimension of the] other as such. (*SVII* 229)

Unable to find the hoped for "good" in oneself, the subject imagines that the Other has it, and fears that, at any point, the Other might take such "goods" away. This scenario results in the tendency to defend one's goods (*défendre ses biens*) which, in Lacan's view, is one and the same thing as "forbidding oneself from enjoying them" (*SVII* 230). Drawing on the double-meaning of the French word "*défendre*", Lacan explains how the sphere of the good "erects a strong wall against the path of desire" (230).[2] In order to cross over said barrier, Lacan conceives his own analytic ethic on the basis of "a radical repudiation of a certain ideal of the good" (230). Whence the significance of Kant for Lacan. Kant took the very thing excluded from the field of traditional ethics and made it the only legitimate territory for ethics. In this way, Kant brought desire into a "pure state". In Seminar XI: *The Four Fundamental Concepts of Psychoanalysis* (1963–1964), Lacan states that, when looked at closely, "Kant's moral law is simply desire in its pure state" which has relevance and cannot be reduced to the logic of the superego (*SXI* 275). Despite his praise, Lacan also criticizes Kant on a number of grounds.

It is noteworthy that Lacan's essay "Kant avec Sade" was intended to serve as a preface to Marquis de Sade's 1795 text *Philosophy of the Bedroom.* With this pairing, Lacan's critique can be summarized in the following way: the best thing Kant had to offer ethics is a kind of *Practical Philosophy* of the Sadean boudoir. Although much has been written on Lacan's notoriously difficult essay, Seminar VII, which preceded it, remains a crucial reference. It is here that Lacan, citing a passage from the *Critique*, argues that "Kant is of the same opinion as Sade" for in order to open the flood gates of desire, both thinkers confront the horizon of pain (*SVII* 80). Taken as the defining principle of the will, Kant claims that the moral law, "by reason of the fact that its sets itself against our inclinations, must produce a feeling that one could call pain" (80). For Kant, pain appears as the only *a priori* feeling that enters into consideration for a rational ethics. Sade's libertines adopt a perverse form of the law: "let us take as the universal maxim of our conduct the right to enjoy any person whatsoever as the instrument of our pleasure" (79). Parallel to the pain endured by Kant's moral subject, access to the Sadean boudoir presumes an intractable pain for those who enter. Lacan thus asserts that:

[2] The play on words in French depends on using "défendre" both in the sense of "defend"—"défendre ses biens"—and "forbid"—"se défendre à soi-même d'en jouir."

> It is enough for [enjoyment] to be a form of evil, for the whole thing to change its character completely, and for the meaning of the moral law itself to be completely changed. Anyone can see that if the moral law is, in effect, capable of playing some role here, it is precisely as support for the enjoyment involved. (*SVII* 189)

As an illustration of Sadean morality, Lacan refers to *Philosophy in the Bedroom* where Sade employs logical arguments to persuade the reader that only "incest, adultery, theft, and everything else you can think of" are in fact the true values of the emerging revolutionary society in France (*KS* 79). The "moral" message of Sade's discourse has the effect of honouring Kant's commitment to rationality as well as his aversion to all "pathological" sentiments. The true world of Kantian ethics is thus envisioned by the cruel and destructive universe enacted by Sade's fantasies. With Sade, Lacan demonstrates that what lies beyond the moral law is a diabolical evil. Instead of happiness, the action of fulfilling the law's prescriptions brings about self-destruction. This suggests, as de Kesel points out, that "enjoyment can no longer be situated inside the limits of desire and the pleasure principle but is to be regarded as an exponent of the death drive" (2009, 125). In following its aim and the laws to which it responds, Lacan explains that desire now serves as an instrument of a transgressive enjoyment: "without transgression, there is no enjoyment" (*SVII* 208).

The search for desire in ethics indicates that our relation to the moral law is fundamentally libidinal. In Sade's boudoir, as in Kantian ethics, the outcome is the same; the striving to satisfy desire can only be experienced in pain. The subject experiences the object of desire negatively in pain due to the impossibility of ever reaching it. This is precisely the limit at which the problematic of desire is raised—and perhaps, realized—in analysis. The realization of desire entails recognition that desire is nothing other than an "infinite measure" (Zupančič 2000). The ethics of desire describes a situation in which the subject expresses fidelity to a lost enjoyment; unable to find the one true object, the subject rejects all other objects and satisfies herself with none. This scenario, illustrated in Lacan's discussion of Antigone, shows how a bearable pain caused by an unfulfilled desire can offer protection against a completely unbearable pain implied by a truly satisfied desire. Although Sade's discourse has the benefit of exposing the radical evil that lies beyond the moral law, he does not conclude that we must keep our distance from this real. Sade's hero makes it his ethical duty to go beyond the law to which he is destructively bound in order to carry out his perverse fantasies while disavowing the pain.

In an effort to formulate the moral consequences of the polymorphous perverse origins of desire, Lacan makes a decisive break with traditional ethics; he claims that, paradoxically, the real "substrate" of the ethically functioning psychic apparatus lies beyond the good in a radical evil (*SVII* 34). For Lacan, enjoyment is what gives ethics its real weight since it allows for the "the meaning of the moral law to be completely changed" (189). In the final analysis, the message of Seminar VII remains tied to the ethical imperative: do not give up on your desire. Rather than extinguish desire, enjoyment, in certain cases, only heightens it and reaffirms the desire to desire. Desire is certainly not Lacan's last word on the end of analysis. In Seminar XI: *The Four Fundamental Concepts of Psychoanalysis* (1963–1963) Lacan begins to link the end of analysis to the concept of the drive: "after the mapping of the subject in relation to the fundamental fantasy, the experience of the [*objet a*] becomes the drive" (*SXI* 273). The shift from desire to drive enacts a supplementary step which Kant, in Lacan's view, failed to take. It also coincides with a theoretical change in Lacan's conception of the status of enjoyment.

In *Ethics of the Real*, Alenka Zupančič explains that, for early Lacan, "[enjoyment] does not exist" or, more precisely, "it exists only in its own loss [...] as something lacking" (2000, 240). This conception, in which the accent is placed on lack and the impossible is identified with the inaccessible, suggests that the end of analysis coincides with the moment when the subject accepts his or her symbolic castration. If the entire pleasure economy rests on an irreducible lack, then enjoyment names the experience that allows the subject to imagine that its lack is overcome. According to Zupančič this is precisely what the notion of the drive is aiming at: a definition of the status of enjoyment as "one-lack-less" (242). This does not mean that the lack is gone. Lacan allows for the subject to cancel out the lack within the symbolic and imaginary registers while remaining marked by it at the level of the real. In this way, Lacan shows how enjoying the desired object is possible. Replacing an earlier insistence on the fidelity to desire's non-satisfaction, Lacan's later work acquires an ethical significance in the call to identify with the drive's senseless satisfaction. Dylan Evans explains that, for Lacan:

> The purpose of the drive (*Triebziel*) is not to reach a *goal* (a final destination) to follow its aim (the way itself), which is to circle round the object [...] Thus the real purpose of the drive is not some mythical goal of full satisfaction, but to return to its circular path, and the real source of enjoyment is the repetitive movement of this closed circuit. (1996, 47)

Lacan's shift from desire to drive raises further questions when we consider his claim, vis-à-vis Freud, that every drive is virtually a *death drive* since it is excessive, repetitive, and ultimately destructive (*KS* 848). While it is beyond the scope of the current section to provide a detailed account of Lacan's use of the concept, it is important to insist on the fact that his later work associates the drive with the notion of the Real as that which resists incorporation into our ordinary experience of reality. In this respect, Slavoj Žižek argues that the whole of Lacan's effort "is precisely focused on those limit-experiences in which the subject finds himself confronted with the death drive at its purest, prior to its reversal into sublimation" (2000, 160). In contrast with his seminar on ethics in which enjoyment could only be reached through transgression of the law, Lacan's presentation of the theory of the four discourses in *The Other Side of Psychoanalysis* (1969–1970) articulates enjoyment together with the signifier. Bearing this in mind, I turn now to Lacan's formulation of contemporary ethics in the 1970s.

6.3 The Event of Speech

In this section, I consider the shift from an ethic focused on how to act to one focused on how to speak. Beginning with Lacan, I approach his discussion of the *éthique du bien-dire* in the 1970s from the perspective of his earlier distinction between full and empty speech. I illustrate these terms through reference to Lacan's L-Schema in order to highlight the imaginary and symbolic dimensions of language. This schema enables me to grasp Lacan's understanding of the psychoanalytic act and the symbolic relations involved in it. I then introduce Lacan's formulation of the *éthique du bien-dire* as an ethic relative to discourse. Focusing on the Analyst's discourse, I describe the *bien-dire* as an ethic that is correlated with the speaking subject which does not dictate behaviors or modes of actions according to universal precepts.

Turning my focus to Foucault, I discuss his analysis of the ancient Greek and Hellenistic concept of *parrhesia* as an ethic of truthful speech. I understand the practice of *parrhesia* to demonstrate the reflexivity of the speaker toward their own position of enunciation. I explain this in terms of the pact that the speaking subject makes with him or herself at the level of the statement and the enunciation. I emphasize the freedom of the declarative pact as involving dangers and risks for the speaker. I differentiate the *parrhesiastic* game from other models of truth-telling to the extent that it entails the struggle over truthfulness in the form of courage, resolve, and endurance rather than a truth that sets one free. I consider the possibility for *parrhesia* to function as a critical relay and apparatus within power relations that challenges paradigmatic figures of authority associated with the rise of disciplinary power. Crucially, I argue that Foucault aligns *parrhesia* with a tradition of critical philosophy that concerns the ontology of the present and the conditions of possibility of the subject's ethical transformations.

6.3.1 The Function of "I" in the *Éthique du bien-dire*

In the 1970s, Lacan shifts the emphasis of psychoanalytic ethics from the question of acting, "have you acted in accordance with your desire?", to the question of speech which now becomes an "*éthique du bien-dire*" (an ethic of the well-spoken) (*T* 65). The aim of psychoanalytic treatment is to lead the analysand to articulate the truth about desire. Here, "truth", is always singular; it is not a single universal truth but a thoroughly particular truth, unique to each subject. For Lacan, truth can only be said partially (*mi-dire*); it is impossible to articulate the whole truth.[3] In *Television*

[3] Lacan states in *Television* "I always tell the truth, not the whole truth because we are incapable of telling it all. Telling it all is materially impossible", p. 9.

(1974), Lacan claims therefore that truth aspires to the Real; "it is related to the real but by the impossible-to-say" (*T* xxni). In Lacan's formulation, the Real is always *trou-matique*; it is a hole in discourse which cannot be said but about which one must speak. Similarly, an ethic of the well-spoken does not dictate behaviors or modes of acting according to universal precepts. Rather, it is a question of approaching the symptom as a subjective manifestation. In this sense, the ethic of the well-spoken can be shown to relate to the implication of the subject in the enjoyment that his/her symptom denounces.[4]

The shift from action to speech is less an opposition of terms than a difference of emphasis since, for Lacan, to speak well is itself an act (Evans 1996). The activity of speaking recalls the historical beginnings of psychoanalysis. In their *Studies on Hysteria* (1895) Breuer and Freud theorized that hysteria is caused by a traumatic event (e.g., sexual abuse) in which repressed emotional reactions were thought to generate hysterical symptomatology. Observed in the case of Bertha Pappenheim, the "talking cure" is a process in which the patient's "talking" removes the blockage of a pathogenic affect resulting, eventually, in a cathartic purgation. For Lacan, the act of speaking in analysis has significance as a symbolic process which is full of signifiers, utterances, and meaning. The focus for Lacan is language itself, which is the site of the unconscious and perhaps, too, the site of a speech act. In the "The Guiding Principles for Any Psychoanalytic Act", a paper presented at the World Association of Psychoanalysis (WAP) in 2004, Eric Laurent, Lacan's former student, presents the first principle in the following way:

> Psychoanalysis is a practice of speech. It involves two partners, the analyst and the analysand, brought together in a single psychoanalytic session. The analysand speaks about what brings him there, his suffering, his symptom. This symptom is hooked into the materiality of the unconscious, made out of things that have been said to the subject, that have hurt him, and things that are impossible to say and cause him suffering.[5]

[4] To recall, Lacan's concept of *jouissance* (enjoyment) expresses the paradoxical satisfaction that the subject derives from his/her symptom, or rather, the suffering s/he derives from satisfaction.

[5] Laurent's text is available at: https://www.lacan.com/ericlaurent.html. [Accessed on 14 March 2021.]

One way to approach the notion of an ethic of the well-spoken is to consider Lacan's earlier distinction between "full speech" and "empty speech" in the psychoanalytic realization of the subject (*ÉS* 30). Lacan's first reference to these terms is found in "The Function and the Field of Speech and Language in Psychoanalysis" (1953). Drawing on Martin Heidegger's conception of linguistic communication developed in the sections on *Rede* (discourse) and *Gerede* (idle chatter) in *Being and Time* (1927), Lacan elaborates his own distinction between *parole pleine* (full speech), and *parole vide* (empty speech). For Lacan, empty speech articulates the imaginary dimension of language where it is linked with "narcissism" and the "illusion of autonomy" (254). Full speech, on the other hand, articulates the symbolic dimension of language which Lacan associates with subject's desire and truth. Unlike empty speech in which the subject talks "about someone in vain [...] who can never become one with the assumption of his desire", full speech targets the opening of a symbolic relational domain (45). In Seminar I: *Freud's Papers on Technique* (1953–1954) Lacan states that:

> Full speech is speech which aims at, which forms, the truth such as it becomes established in the recognition of one person by another. Full speech is speech which performs [*qui fait acte*]. (*SI* 107)

Lacan employs "full" and "empty" speech in the context of analytic treatment to designate extreme points on a continuum during which the analyst listens to the analysand. In the secondary literature, empty speech is often portrayed as both a necessary condition for and impediment to the event of full speech. Philippe Julien (1994) understands the imaginary dimension of communication to constitute an impasse which is inherent to intersubjective exchange and not merely an anomaly which arises in everyday speech and blocks true dialogue. Collette Soler (1996) holds that empty speech offers a means of connecting with others in that it calls out for the recognition that others can provide which is nonetheless insufficient for transformation. Derek Hook (2013) refers empty speech to the imaginary axis of one-to-one intersubjective dialogue and behavior that serves the ego and functions to consolidate the images subjects use to substantiate themselves. Empty speech thus conveys the notion that the act of speaking holds out the potential for truth but brings with it the trappings of illusion.

The imaginary domain of empty speech describes a type of exchange which locks each participant into the narcissistic closed circuit of ego-led speech. Providing an example of one such ego-to-ego interaction, Hook recalls a scene from the American TV series *The Sopranos* which takes place between Tony and his replacement therapist who listens to Tony's stories and responds with his ego. Hook thus describes a situation "where two speakers, seemingly involved in a dialogue, are actually involved in two self-enclosed monologues, each using the other as the mute audience to a story they are telling themselves about themselves" (2013, 8). Empty speech is a way of shoring up or lending consistency to the ego whereby talking takes on the illusory status of an autonomous project of self-making. In the context of the psychoanalytic realization of the subject—the Lacanian notion that the subject "speaks" him or herself into existence–, empty speech enables belief in the "substantial" entity that we invoke.

The notion of empty speech establishes a crucial proviso for thinking about the "talking cure" inasmuch as it shows how talk is continually conditioned by the tendency on the part of both speakers to affirm the ego, to protect and shield it against what it considers harmful, and to mobilize its defenses against hearing anything which might be too unsettling. Despite being a necessary precondition for discourse at all, empty speech underscores the inherent challenges of communication: it shows that the speaking subject is typically more concerned with upholding an ideal image of its ego and gaining the recognition of others, than with what the message communicates per se. For its part, psychoanalysis remains suspicious of anything which gratifies the ego's inherent narcissism or provides it with a comforting image of itself and the world, since this necessarily involves a move away from reality or, rather, the Real.

In the 1950s Lacan begins to introduce schemata into his work in an attempt to formalize certain aspects of psychoanalytic theory. The L Schema (Fig. 6.1) serves as a means of mapping both the dialogue between two subjects as well as the description of distinct points that constitute

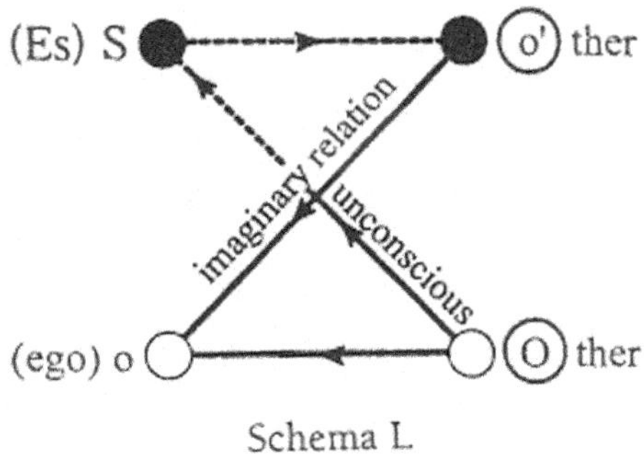

Fig. 6.1 Lacan's L Schema

the subject's singular subjectivity.[6] For this reason, the L schema is often explained in terms of its intersubjective relations and intrasubjective structure. The diagram depicts two facets of the individual, <S> (subject) and <o> (ego), located on the left-hand side that converse with another ego <o'>, situated on the upper right-hand side. The interaction between the ego and the other brings into play another principle of Otherness <O>, depicted on the lower right-hand side. The presence of a third point of reference indicates that dialogue must be grounded in something other than the standpoints of its two participants and their ego-led speech. The name given to this third position—which functions, as an amalgamation of social conventions and laws, as the embodiment of authority—is the Big Other (Žižek 1989, 1992; Fink 1995).

For Lacan, the L Schema represents "the interruption of full speech between the subject and the Other and its detour through the two egos, o and o', and their imaginary relations" (*SIII* 14). The schema helps convey the notion that the symbolic relation between the Other and the subject <O—S> is always blocked, to a certain extent, by the imaginary axis between the ego and other <o'—o>. The Other-subject relation <O—S>, linked by the diagonal that bisects the imaginary axis, designates the symbolic axis of communication. In contrast to ego-to-ego speech, the symbolic axis refers to the way in which the subject <S>

[6] Regarding this last point, Lacan states that the "[subject] is stretched over the four corners of the schema" and not merely located at the mark designated <S>, p. 459.

communicates within a given socio-symbolic context by utilizing the codes, signifiers and language supplied by the Other, <O>. For an "interruption" to occur there must be something Other in the subject's speech, something which speaks "beyond" the subject and seems not to have been said by the subject or adequately integrated into the field of one's conscious ego identity. Discussing the role of free association in clinical analysis, which operates without conscious control, Lacan claims that it opens onto "full speech which is painful to [the speaking subject]" (*ÉS* 193).[7]

In place of the comfort and reassurance of empty speech, full speech aims to undo the identifications that provide the basis for the subject's ego. For Lacan, the "interruption of full speech between the subject and the Other" serves not only to provoke anxiety in the subject, but also to disrupt the operations of ego-led speech, thus providing a means for symbolic mediation and communicative change (*SIII* 14). For change to occur in analysis, the subject must first traverse the fantasy which Bruce Fink describes as a process of separation that involves "subjectifying one's fate, that foreign cause (the Other's desire) that brought one into existence" (*PU* 79).[8] Applied to Lacan's formula of the fantasy, <$ ◊ *a*>, this traversing means that the subject crosses the lozenge and assumes the cause of its own advent.[9] Fink refers the traversal of the fantasy to a utopian moment beyond the castration complex which, "unlike other utopian moments (e.g., 'full speech')", was never recanted in Lacan's later work to his knowledge (*PU* 79). Fink's comments have the benefit of shifting our discussion from Lacan's notion of full speech to his formulation of the *éthique du bien-dire* in the 1970s.

---

[7] See Lacan's text "The Direction of the Treatment and the Principles of its Powers" (1961) included as part of the 2001 volume *Écrits: A Selection,* translated by Alan Sheridan, pp. 173–214.

[8] It is perhaps helpful here to recall our discussion in 6.2.2 where we linked the "domain of the goods" to the "desire of the Other". In Lacanian theory, in order for the libidinal being to become a subject s/he must first assume the desire of the Other. Traversing the fantasy describes the point at which the subject subjectifies the Other's desire and assumes a new position in relation to the cause.

[9] The discussion in 6.2.2 also linked the traversal of the fantasy to the end of analysis and to the concept of the drive: "after mapping the subject in relation to the *a* the experience of the fundamental fantasy becomes the drive" (1978, 273).

In a filmed dialogue with Jacques-Alain Miller which was partially transcribed and later published under the title *Television: A Challenge to the Psychoanalytic Establishment*, Lacan was asked to respond to the Kantian question "What should I do?". To this Lacan replies: "I can only take up the question as anyone else would, by posing it to myself [a]nd the reply is simple [i]t is what I am doing, deriving from my practice the ethic of the well-spoken" (*T* 41). Discussing his own practice, Lacan describes how psychoanalytic experience passes through a structure of discourse which concerns the way the singular unconscious of each subject follows the social link. The implication is that "an ethic is relative to a discourse" in general and to the Discourse of the Analyst in particular (*T* 42). In the 1950s, Lacan conceives the analyst as a stand-in for the Big Other <A>. At this level, the function of the analyst is to frustrate the subject's imaginary misrecognitions and to make the subject accept their place in the circuit of symbolic exchange.[10] In Seminar XVII (1969–1970) Lacan positions the analyst as a stand-in for the analysand's *objet petit a*, illustrated in the schema <*a* → $>.

Here the function of the analyst is to demonstrate that the *objet a* is produced by its very exclusion from discourse: it is desired precisely because it is missing. By standing-in for that which is missing, the analyst is uniquely positioned to confront desire with its own phantasmatic support. For this reason, Lacan states that the Discourse of the Analyst "enables fantasy to resurface in a completely balanced way" (*SXVII* 108). In analysis, the subject comes to recognize the object s/he had been for the Other. What remains of this object after traversing the fantasy is a hole (*trou*) and it is around this hole that the structure of discourse revolves. The social link of the Analyst enables the subject to confront the structural lack in the Other and correlatively in oneself. By remaining at the level of the castrated subject, the subject continues to be plagued by the Other's desire while obtaining a secondary gain from his or her symptomatic submission to the Other. For Lacan, the ethic of the well-spoken

[10] In Seminar III (1993), Lacan states "if one wants to position the analyst within this schema of the subject's speech, one can say that he is somewhere in <A>" p. 161.

is correlated with the implication of the speaking subject in the enjoyment that his symptom denounces.[11]

With his neologism *jouis-sens*, Lacan foregrounds the satisfaction derived from surplus meaning. The hysterical subject exemplifies this type of satisfaction by asking the Other to assign a meaning to the riddle s/he poses while exposing, in turn, the deficiencies inherent in every given meaning. To this the analyst responds with silence in order to point out the "flaw" in meaning insofar as it aims at more meaning, *plus-de-sens*. Rather demanding signifiers from the Other, the Analyst prompts the subject to produce his or her own. Situated in the place of discursive product, Lacan refers to the <S1> in the Discourse of the Analyst as *la bêtise*. Stressing the centrality of free association, Lacan reiterates that the goal of psychoanalysis is not to "say it all", but to say whatever comes to mind without worrying about saying something stupid. Variously translated in English as "funny business" and "little stupidity", *la bêtise* speaks more powerfully and immediately to unconscious material than those things that we consciously intend to say.[12] If the ethic of the well-spoken aims at full speech, it is perhaps a speech full of double meanings and equivocation from which the analyst creates a space in which sense-enjoyment (*jouis-sens*) no longer has any meaning for the speaking subject.

To grasp the way the subject "speaks" itself into being in analysis, Lacan distinguishes between the grammatical "I" of the statement and the unconscious "I" of the enunciation. In the *Ethics of the Real*, Alenka Zupančič states that contrary to the proper noun which has the function of filling the gap in the Other, the "I" opens an irreparable void: "[it] disables the battery of signifiers, and makes [them] in-complete, *pas toute*; for it is an element [...] that refers to something outside the linguistic structure: to the act of speech itself" (2000, 30). Whereas the subject of the statement is determined in advance by the given signifiers, the subject of the enunciation, defined in relation to the shifter "I", is determined retroactively. In Seminar XI (1963–1964), Lacan says of the shifter "I"

[11] See Daniela Chatelard's article « Du bien-dire et du réel dans la psychanalyse », Psychanalyse, 2016/1 (n° 35), pp. 39–45.

[12] In *The Lacanian Subject* (1995) Fink suggests "funny business", arguing that *la bêtise* "is a piece of nonsense produced by the analytic process itself", p. 135.

that it becomes "a signification, engendered at the level of the statement, of what it produces at the level of enunciation" or, at the level of something which becomes what "it is" in the act of speaking itself (*SXI* 139). Although the subject of the act is never fully transparent to itself or aware of what it wants, Zupančič argues that:

> [T]he subject is "realized", "objectified" in this act: the subject passes over to the side of the object. The ethical subject is not a subject who wants this object but, rather, this object itself. In an act, there is no "divided subject": there is the "it". (2000, 104)

The "object" in question can be perhaps linked to the object of the drive, with the Analyst's discourse facilitating the subject's encounter with the drive <*a* → $>. In the 1970s, following the shift in the end of analysis from desire to drive, Lacan concedes that there is no ethic beside that of the *éthique du bien-dire* (*T* 22). The duty of the well-spoken is "to find one's way in dealing with the unconscious, with the structure" (22). Because psychoanalysis is unable to create an alternative ethical law through its discourse, it cannot offer a critique of ethics in the traditional sense. The practice of psychoanalysis as an ethic of the well-spoken can only decenter ethics. On one hand, this decentering brings into play the Freudian scandal of a polymorphous perversion, on the other hand, it takes place in the divided speaking subject who is deprived of any substantial content.

6.3.2 Fearless Truth-Telling

In this section, I introduce Foucault's discussions on the ethical practice of ancient *parrhesia*. Foucault's analysis of the notion of *parrhesia*, which began in 1982 and continued in 1983 during his lecture course "The Government of Self and Others", develops a specific model of truth-telling that transforms the *ethos* of its interlocutor, carries certain risks for the speaker, and belongs to a temporality of present reality. With the Greek and Hellenistic concept of *parrhesia* Foucault finds that true discourse need not be taken up through the wonted lens of the analytic of truth. Forms of truth-telling could be placed within the framework of a critical ontology in order to analyze the different modes of being that true discourses entail for the subject who uses them. In "The Courage of Truth" (1983–1984) Foucault refers to this as the study of "alethurgic forms" or acts by which truth is manifested to differentiate the analysis of the subject's ethical transformations from the analysis of epistemological structures (*CT* 3).

My entry into *parrhesia* begins from the premise that it is an act of speech which has the function of enacting the speaker's relationship to truth and the reflexivity which the speaker demonstrates toward their own position of enunciation. Foucault explains in various ways that the *parrhesiastic* utterance not only transmits some content, but simultaneously, conveys the way the speaker relates to this content. In *Fearless Speech*, Foucault asserts that "in parrhesia the speaker emphasizes the fact that he is both the subject of the enunciation and the subject of the *enunciandum*—that he himself is the opinion to which he refers" (*FS* 13). This idea is further elaborated in "The Government of Self and Others" where Foucault claims that *parrhesia* "includes the statement of the truth, and then, on top of this statement, an implicit element which could be called the *parrhesiastic* pact of the subject with himself, by which he binds himself to the content of the statement and to the act of making it" (*GSO* 65).

In "The Government of Self and Others" Foucault presents *parrhesia* within an ethics of self-transformation: "in producing the event of the [*parrhesiastic*] utterance, the subject modifies, or affirms, or anyway determines and clarifies his mode of being insofar as he speaks" (*GSO* 68). The speaker therefore says something, declares oneself the one who said it, and on the basis of this declarative statement, brings about something new. Subjective transformation occurs at the moment of the declaration, not at the moment of what the speaker goes on to do. Citing the example of Plato at Syracuse confronting the tyrant, Dionysius, Foucault insists that "there is *parrhesia* from the moment Plato actually accepts the risk of being exiled, killed, sold," in telling the truth (67). The methodological context in which Foucault situates his analysis of *parrhesia* describes a scenario where "true discourse determines an open situation [...] and makes possible effects which are, precisely, not known" (63). To further emphasize this point, Foucault contrasts the analysis of *parrhesia* with that of the performative utterance:

> [Parrhesia] is the opposite of the performative, in which the enunciation of something brings about and gives rise to a completely determined event as a function of the general code and institutional field in which the utterance is made. Here, on the contrary, it is a truth-telling, an irruptive truth-telling which creates a fracture and opens up the risk: a possibility, a field of dangers, or at any rate, an undefined eventuality. (67)

Parrhesia, in other words, announces those truths which radically destabilize the present by transforming the way being itself is interpreted. Foucault is careful not to define the "truth" of *parrhesiastic* speech, he emphasizes instead the extent to which *parrhesia* opens up an interference and dissonance with the present in order to instantiate an altered, unknowable future. Rather than trying to represent a political or social state of affairs as it is, *parrhesia* constitutes an "irruptive event" within discourse which allows for transformative sayings without themselves stating the *whole* truth. For those involved in the *parrhesiastic* game, *parrhesia* provides a means to introduce a new field of social relations in which the *parrhesiastes* and the listener may begin to operate. In its relay to others, Edward McGushin notes that *parrhesiastic* engagement is often risky and "painful" (2007, 7). This is because *parrhesia* has the function of enacting disruptive truths which threaten the listener's comfortable position in life and demand a new responsibility. Foucault describes the *parrhesiastes*, unlike the rhetorician (who persuades) or the flatterer (who charms), as a courageous truth-teller who puts himself and his relationship with others at an unspecified risk:

> For there to be parrhesia [...] the subject must be taking some kind of risk [in speaking] this truth which he signs as his opinion, his thought, his belief, a risk which concerns his relationship with the person to whom he is speaking [...] in speaking the truth one must open up, establish, and confront the risk of offending the other person, of irritating him, of making him angry and provoking him to conduct which may even be extremely violent. (*FS* 11)

Foucault is careful not to situate the *parrhesiastes* in an abstract, ethereal realm of truth; the *parrhesiastes* does not live in philosophic solitude apart from others. The relationship with the Other is therefore a basic condition for *parrhesiastic* speech. In its extreme form, Foucault states that the *parrhesiastic* game takes place between "the threat of death [which] comes from the Other" and "the security of life where the truth goes unspoken" (*FS* 17). Socrates' fate at the end of Plato's *Apology* illustrates the life-threatening stakes of the game. To merit consideration as a *parrhesiastes* there must be a risk of danger in telling the truth. In *Fearless Speech*, Foucault explains that danger is intensified by the fact that "parrhesia comes from 'below', as it were, and is directed toward 'above'" (18). *Parrhesia* always occurs in situations where the speaker is in a position of inferiority with respect to the interlocutor. To summarize these points, then, the truth of *parrhesiastic* speech is produced and sustained within power relations not outside them where truth is made to function as a critical apparatus and relay.

In her article "Truthfulness, Risk and Trust in the Late Lectures of Michel Foucault" (1994), Nancy Luxon argues that Foucault finds in ancient practices of *parrhesia* a resource by which to evaluate modern authorities that claim to speak truthfully and derive their authority from this claim. Luxon proposes a three-tier analytic framework to show how Foucault develops a powerful model of truth-telling which does not "require the audience to have more or better access to truth, to have any specialized knowledge, or to be in a position to trump the claims of the speaker" (1994, 483). Seen from this angle, the *parrhesiastes* is contrasted with the figure of the modern expert who perpetuates the dynamic that binds power and knowledge together. Foucault's model of truth-telling fashions these authorities along new lines that eventually generates bonds of trust between the speaker and the audience. With the emphasis on risk and danger, Foucault places *parrhesia* within the coordinates of a critical speech that urges us to interrogate politics rather than asking questions that already belong to a political doctrine.

Foucault presents *parrhesia* as an ethic of truthful speech that helps to modify both the speaker's and the listener's relationship to truth. Yet without the difficulty of the challenge of the *parrhesiastic game* and the possibility of overextending beyond the game's limits, real change is not possible. In the "Government and Self and Others", Foucault focuses his analysis of parrhesia on the question: "how is the obligation of truth [...] the exercise of freedom and the dangerous exercise of freedom?" (*GSO* 67). Foucault argues that *parrhesia* appears only in an agonistic field where it relates to rivalry, conflict, and confrontation. In contrast to later Enlightenment projects of subject-formation, Luxon claims that "neither the truth-claims nor the self-examination that result from this engagement will set the participant free" (1994, 474). Foucault's model valorizes not a liberatory truth but a process of struggle in which freedom is something to be exercised rather than attained. The *parrhesiastes* is aware of the risks s/he accepts and recognizes that his or her interlocutor might transgress the limits of the game through recourse to violence. In this way, the *parrhesiastes* uses his or her freedom to risk a declarative pact with truth and him or herself which tests the boundaries of the game's rules with all its consequences rather than making use of those rules to reproduce her own authority.

Parrhesiastic speech must therefore establish the vulnerability of each person in order to transform them. The dynamic of the game is processual; as it unfolds, it allows others and oneself to see the truth in bare form. For Foucault, the *parrhesiastes* is someone who does not hide anything, rather "he opens his heart and mind completely to other people through his discourse" (*FS* 12). This is particularly evident in the context of ancient spiritual direction, as explored in Plato's *Gorgias*, where Foucault captures the emotional and psychic bond between *parrhesiastes* and interlocutor, as well as the relationship's pedagogical structure. With his term "psychagogy", Foucault describes a relationship that is based on an intellectual and emotional affinity that ranges from friendship to eroticism. The affective tie which binds the listener to the speaker is necessary for *parrhesia* to have the function of modifying the mode of being of the addressee. Here, Foucault presents *parrhesia* within the pre-history of the practices that developed around the famous couples of penitent-confessor and analyst-analysand. Unlike Christian spirituality, however, Foucault claims that in Greco-Roman Antiquity the obligation of (*parrhesiastic*) truth falls on the side of the spiritual guide:

> In Greco-Roman philosophy, the person who must be present within the true discourse is the person who guides. And he does not have to be present in the form of the utterance's reference [...] and he is not present as the person who says: "This is what I am." He is present in a coincidence between the subject of enunciation and the subject of his own actions. "This truth I tell you, you see it in me.". (*HoS* 409)

Foucault carefully distinguishes between speaking *for* others and speaking *with* others. In grounding the authority of the *parrhesiastes*, Foucault stresses that such a role develops contextually and is not delimited by an institutionalized position: the *parrhesiastes* is "not a professional" (*HoS* 155). The authoritative positions of *parrhesiastes* are more fluidly and variously structured than those of the Christian spiritual director or the modern "expert". The *parrhesiastes* could be a pedagogue, a friend, a lover, or all three. A central question in Foucault's ethic, as John Rajchman observes, is the importance of community which concerns the bonds that we can have with one another, whether affective or political (1991, 99). Beyond the spiritual bond which ties the speaker to the listener, Foucault reminds us that the *parrhesiastes* "primarily chooses a specific relationship to himself" (2001, 17). As Foucault indicates at the outset of his 1983 course, the concept of *parrhesia* is implicated within a bundle of important notions that include "care of self, knowledge of self, art and exercise of oneself" (*GSO* 45). This suggests that *parrhesia* is not only critical to political and pedagogical relations with others, but also to self-reflexive forms of resistance and the stylization of one's existence.

Foucault's analysis of parrhesia aligns with his specific aim of writing a history of a different kind of critical philosophy that concerns the conditions and undefined possibilities of the subject's transformation. This entails an exercise of freedom which results in the ability to speak for oneself rather than to defer to others who are ready to speak on one's behalf. It is worth pointing out that in the "Government of Self and Others" Foucault situates Kant's text on *Aufklärung* as a sort of prolegomenon to the study of ancient *parrhesia* as an ethical practice thus enacting a crucial shift in his own discursive positioning. The threat that connects Foucault with the Enlightenment is an ethico-political task described as the reactivation of a limit-attitude: "an ethos, a philosophical life in which the critique of what we are is at one and the same time the historical analysis of the limits imposed on us and an experiment with the possibility of going beyond them" (2007, 132). Foucault's project of a critical ontology of ourselves arguably begins with the pact of the speaking subject in the act of truth-telling.

References

Breuer, J., & Freud, S. (1974) *Studies on Hysteria*. Harmondsworth: Penguin Books.

De Kesel, M. (2009) *Eros and Ethics: Reading Jacques Lacan's Seminar VII*. Albany: SUNY Press.

Deleuze, G., Guattari, F. (1983) *Anti-Oedipus: Capitalism and Schizophrenia*. Translated from the French by R. Hurley, M. Seem, H. R. Lane. Minneapolis: University of Minnesota Press.

Evans, D. (1996) *An Introductory Dictionary of Lacanian Psychoanalysis*. New York/London: Routledge.

Fink, B. (1995) *The Lacanian Subject between Language and Jouissance*. New Jersey: Princeton University Press.

Foucault, M. (1982) "The Subject and Power", *Critical Inquiry*, 8(4), pp. 777–795. Available at: http://www.jstor.org/stable/1343197 [Accessed: 27 January 2021]

Foucault, M. (1986) "A Preface to Transgression", in Bouchard, F. & Simon, S. (eds.) *Language, Counter-Memory, Practice: Selected Essays and Interviews*. New York: Cornell University Press. (1977b, pp. 29–52).

Foucault, M. (1990) *The History of Sexuality, Volume 2: The Use of Pleasure*. Translated from the French by R. Hurley. New York: Vintage Books.

Foucault, M. (1997) *Ethics: Subjectivity and Truth*, Paul Rabinow (ed.). Translated from the French by R. Hurley and others. New York: New Press.

Foucault, M. (2001) *Fearless Speech*, Pearson, J. (ed.). Translated from the French by J. Pearson. Los Angeles: Semiotext(e).

Foucault, M. (2005) *The Hermeneutics of the Subject: Lectures at the Collège de France 1981–1982*, Gros, F. (ed.). Translated from the French by G. Burchell. New York: Palgrave Macmillan.

Foucault, M. (2007) *The Politics of Truth*, Lotringer, S. (ed.). Translated from the French by L. Hochroth & C. Porter. Los Angeles: Semiotext(e).

Foucault, M. (2008) *Psychiatric Power: Lectures at the Collège de France, 1973–1974*, Lagrange, J. (ed.). Translated from the French by G. Burchell. New York: Picador.

Foucault, M. (2010a) *The Government of Self and Others: Lectures at the Collège de France, 1982–1983*, Gros, F. (ed.). Translated from the French by G. Burchell. New York: Palgrave Macmillan.

Foucault, M. (2010b) *The Birth of Biopolitics: Lectures at the Collège de France, 1978–1979*, Senellart, M. (ed.). Translated from the French by G. Burchell. New York: Palgrave Macmillan.

Foucault, M.. (2011) *The Courage of Truth (the Government of Self and Others II): Lectures at the Collège de France, 1983–1984*, Gros, F. (ed.). Translated from the French by G. Burchell. New York: Palgrave Macmillan.

Hook, D. (2013) "Nixon's 'full-speech': Imaginary and Symbolic Registers of Communication", *Journal of Theoretical and Philosophical Psychology*, 33 (1), pp. 32–50.

Julien, P. (1994) *Jacques Lacan's Return to Freud the Real, the Symbolic and the Imaginary*. New York and London: New York University Press.

Lacan, J. (1966) "Kant avec Sade" *in Écrits*. Paris: Editions du Seuil, pp. 763–92.

Lacan, J. (1978) *The Seminar of Jacques Lacan, Book XI: The Four Fundamental Concepts of Psychoanalysis*, J. A. Miller (ed.). Translated from the French by A. Sheridan. New York/London: W. W. Norton & Company.

Lacan, J. (1988) *The Seminar of Jacques Lacan, Book I: Freud's Papers on Technique, 1953–1954*, J. A. Miller (ed.). Translated from the French by J. Forrester. Cambridge: Cambridge University Press.

Lacan, J. (1990) *Television: A Challenge to the Psychoanalytic Establishment*, J. Copjec (ed.). Translated from the French by D. Hollier. New York/London: W. W. Norton & Company.

Lacan, J. (1992) *The Seminar of Jacques Lacan*, Book VII: The Ethics of Psychoanalysis, J. A. Miller (ed.). Translated from the French by D. Porter. New York/London: W.W. Norton & Company.

Lacan, J. (1993) *The Seminar of Jacques Lacan, Book III: The Psychoses, 1955–1956*, J. A. Miller (ed.). Translated from the French by R. Grigg. New York/London: W. W. Norton & Company.

Lacan, J. (1995) "The Position of the Unconscious", in R. Feldstein, B. Fink, & M. Jaanus (eds.) *Reading Seminar XI: Lacan's Four Fundamental Concepts of Psychoanalysis*. Translated from the French by B. Fink. Albany: SUNY Press, pp. 259–277.

Lacan, J. (2001) *Écrits: A Selection.* Translated from the French by A. Sheridan. London: Routledge.

Lacan, J. (2007) *The Seminar of Jacques Lacan, Book XVII: The Other Side of Psychoanalysis, 1969–1970,* Miller, J. A. (ed.). Translated from the French by R. Grigg. New York: W.W. Norton and Company.

Lazzarato, M. (2002) "From Biopower to Biopolitics", *Pli,* 13, pp. 99–113.

Luxon, N. (1994) "Truthfulness, Risk, and Trust in the Late Lectures of Michel Foucault", *Inquiry: An Interdisciplinary Journal of Philosophy,* 47 (5), pp. 464–489.

Mcgushin, E. (2007) *Foucault's Askesis: An Introduction to the Philosophical Life.* Evanston: Northwestern University Press.

Rajchman, J. (1991) *Truth and Eros: Foucault, Lacan and the Question of Ethics.* New York/London: Routledge.

Read, J. (2009) "A Genealogy of Homo-Economicus: Neoliberalism and the Production of Subjectivity", *Foucault Studies,* 6, pp. 25–36.

Soler, C. (1996) "The Symbolic Order (I)", in Feldstein, R., Fink, B., & Jaanus M. (eds.) *Reading Seminars I & II Lacan's return to Freud.* New Jersey: SUNY Press: pp. 39–46.

Žižek, S. (1989) *The Sublime Object of Ideology.* London & New York: Verso.

Žižek, S. (1992) *Looking Awry: An Introduction to Jacques Lacan through Popular Culture.* Cambridge: MIT Press.

Žižek, S. (2000) "Class Struggle or Postmodernism? Yes, please!", in Butler, J., Laclau, E., & Žižek, S. (eds.) *Contingency, Hegemony, Universality.* London: Verso, pp. 90–135.

Zupančič, A.(2000) *The Ethics of the Real: Kant and Lacan.* London/New York: Verso.

7

Conclusion: Toward a New Erotics—Foucault with

7.1 Introduction

This chapter marks the end of Part II "The Analyst" and signals the possibility of thinking Lacan and Foucault together in relation to the question of "erotics" and will effectively conclude this book. The title of the chapter refers to an excerpt from John Rajchman's *Truth and Eros: Foucault, Lacan and the Question of Ethics* in which he argues that both thinkers direct the passion of their thought to an analysis of what, in our experience, exceeds our identifications with our ways of life, opening them to questioning and transformation without the assurance of an ideal on which to model ourselves:

> In this unsettling of our identities would lie the problem of a "new erotics": of a new type of bond not based on the exigencies of the super-ego; or a new type of community based on what we already know ourselves and the ways we have come to govern ourselves. In the "beauty" of our tragic libidos or historical fatalities, would thus lie an attempt to rethink the ancient question of *ethos*: how to be "at home" in a world where our identity is not given, our being-together in question, our destiny contingent or uncertain: the world of the violence of our own self-constitution. (1991, 144)

J. L. Davis, *Reading Foucault Through Lacan*, The Palgrave Lacan Series,
https://doi.org/10.1007/978-3-031-69738-8_7

Rajchman's commentary is useful in that it presents a juncture in which Lacan and Foucault approach the question of subjectivity not in terms of who we *must* be, but how we might live in the world without the supposition of a fundamental or unproblematic identity, or where it becomes the object of analysis. The problem of a "new erotics" is thus one in which "we" ourselves are in question, "we" ourselves whose experience is always departing from our identifications. To re-think subjectivity in this way is to confront the difficulty with ourselves, our freedom with respect to who and what we are said to be, and the bonds of which we are capable. In this chapter, I consider the attempt that both Lacan and Foucault make to invent a new style of thought, a style which belongs to a crisis in contemporary ethics. While I share Rajchman's view that the philosophies of each thinker require a new social form, "not a School with its Master, not a University with its Experts", I go further in suggesting that "erotics" is specific to the social link of the Analyst which, in Lacan's theory, represents a structural inversion of the traditional Master along with its modern discursive mutation (1991, 146).

To this end, I show that Foucault and Lacan are engaged in questions about identity, the forms of bonds we can have with one another, the new sorts of rules we can yet invent, whether an ethical "authority" or "mastery" can even exist, and what it might look like. Chapter 7 is divided into two parts. The first part, Sect. 7.2 "An Affective Encounter", explores the notion of an erotic experience from the preliminary perspective of an intense emotional relationship. Beginning with Lacan in Sect. 7.2.1, "Two Schemas of Love", I first discuss the imaginary dimension in which transference unfolds under the guise of particularly strong affects such as love and hate. I then reflect on Lacan's claim that transference manifests itself first and foremost as the love of knowledge. This allows me to distinguish between two types of love: "romantic" and "Real". I describe the suspension of the field of meaning and the symbolic order by the Analyst as holding the analysand's address for love through an encounter with the Real.

In Sect. 7.2.2 "Two Erotic Domains: Care and Psychagogy" I examine two aspects of the erotic encounter in ancient Greece as analyzed by Foucault in his genealogy of ethics. I show that the domain of erotics functions as a key reference point for the changes that occurred in ethical self-constitution between the Classical era and Late Antiquity. I base my discussion on Foucault's detailed readings of Plato's Socratic dialogues which he presents in his lectures at the Collège de France between 1982 and 1984. Beginning with *Alcibiades I*, I describe how Foucault introduces Socrates as a new kind of lover who cares for the soul of his beloved. This example allows me to demonstrate via the concept of *epimeleia heauton* that knowledge, which is a necessary element of the *care of the self*, is only achieved through an erotic attachment between master and disciple. Shifting the focus to Plato's *Gorgias*, I highlight the *parrhesiastic* function of philosophy as a "psychagogy"; a pedagogy and an erotics that lose their amorous character and become relations of intense *philia*. Foucault understands *parrhesiastic* philosophy in its psychagogic activity not simply as a form of knowledge but a style of discourse which aims at the transformation of the subject(s) who speak and listen.

Through this discussion, I highlight the significance of "erotics" as relations combining pleasure and power between two unequal parties. To illustrate this perspective, I refer to Lacan's Seminar VIII: *Transference* (1960–1961) where he draws on Plato's *Symposium* to thematize the erotic nature of desire from a psychoanalytic point of view. The relation between Socrates and Alcibiades allows me to demonstrate that there is no mutuality between lover and beloved. For Lacan, love is marked by a constitutive dissymmetry and inequality. Similarly, Foucault explains that *epimeleia heauton* was thematized as a response to the limits of Athenian pedagogy and the erotic field which was used as an opportunity for the lover to seduce the beloved who was at a great disadvantage in the erotic game. Alongside other aspects of erotic experience including signification, separation, and differentiation, I consider the relation between erotics and politics insofar as the former leaves open the contestable space of disparity.

I introduce the second part of Chap. 7 under the heading "The Ethics of Eros" where I discuss the attempts that Lacan and Foucault make to re-think eros while reflecting on the way in which the eros of their thought can be linked to ethics. In Sect. 7.3.1 "Foucault: An Erotic Method" I return to John Rajchman who writes of Foucault that perhaps in our eros we are neither Greek nor Christian nor Freudian but are becoming something else. I take this "something else" to be a salient feature of Foucault's ethics which does not tell us who we are or what to do but offers us instead the possibilities of refusal, curiosity and innovation. I present Foucault as an erotic thinker through reference to the method and movement of genealogy which does not take ethics at face value but begins by putting ethical ideals in questions.

Section 7.3.2, "Lacan: The Feminine Knower and Its Discourse", recalls Rajchman's claim that Lacan, by refusing knowledge of a Good or Ideal makes "the eros of our not-knowing the principle of […] a new kind of philosophy" (1991, 26). I raise the parallel question of how to understand the Discourse of the Analyst and the subject position of (not-)knowing it makes available as being sexualized. Through reference to Jeanne Schroeder's *The Four Lacanian Discourses* and Kirsten Campbell's *Jacques Lacan and Feminist Epistemology*, I explain how sexual difference is inscribed in Lacan's matrix of the four discourses. Drawing on Lacan's Seminar XX: *Encore* (1972–1973) I read his graph of sexuation from the masculine side to identify the feminine subject in the position of *non all* which represents both an objection to the phallic signifier and a signification of its limit. I conclude Sect. 7.3 with a general reflection on the discourses of psychoanalysis that signify in excess of what a phallic regime can capture. In reference to Lynne Huffer's *Foucault's Strange Eros*, I describe eros through the lens of an encounter with the work of each thinker and the subjective experience of writing this book.

7.2 An Affective Encounter

In this section, I explore the notion of an erotic experience from the preliminary perspective of an affective encounter with the other. Beginning with Lacan, I discuss the imaginary dimension in which transference often unfolds in analysis under the guise of particularly strong affects such as love and hate. Through reference to Seminar VIII: *Transference* (1960–1961), I consider the significance Lacan attributes to Plato's *Symposium* to illustrate the relationship between analyst and analysand. I reflect on Lacan's view that transference manifests itself, first and foremost, as the love of knowledge. Psychoanalysis, as Lacan understands it, recognizes the supposition of a subject who knows and the eros that underlies it. I describe the way the Lacanian analyst holds the address for knowledge in transference in terms of "real" love. I identify the suspension of the field of meaning and the symbolic order by the analyst as an encounter with the Real by which the analysand changes his or her relationship to knowledge.

Turning to Foucault, I explain that the domain of erotics functions as a key reference point for his genealogy of ethics in ancient Greece and for the changes that occurred in ethical self-constitution between the Classical era and late Antiquity. Through reference to Foucault's lectures at the Collège de France between 1981 and 1983, I consider two aspects of the erotic relation as presented in Foucault's readings of Plato's Socratic dialogues. The first, which I discuss in relation to Plato's *Alcibiades*, brings into focus the transformation of erotics into a practice of care. I understand Foucault's emphasis on the *epimeleia heauton* (care of oneself) to introduce a new dimension into the rather limiting role that eros plays in the traditional acquisition of philosophical knowledge. In the second example, I discuss Plato's *Gorgias* to highlight the parrhesiastic function of philosophical discourse that operates as an intense affective relation between master and disciple. This enables me to underscore the spiritual or transformative function of an encounter with the *parrhesiastes* that is both pedagogic and erotic.

The question "what is an erotic experience" unfolds through my discussions of Lacan and Foucault. Both thinkers start from the premise that erotic relations take place between two unequal parties such as a lover and a beloved or a subject and object. The implication is that the love relationship is always marked by dissymmetry and inequality. In Sect. 7.2.1 "Two Schemas of Love: Romantic and Real", I discuss erotic experience as an initial affective encounter between the analyst and analysand that establishes a context for signification and separation. In Sect. 7.2.2, "Two Erotic Domains: Care and Psychagogy", I link erotic experience to the issue of being sexed in corporeal intimate relations between adult and adolescent males in ancient Greece. These examples enable me to foreground the experience of differentiation in which something takes place that changes the two beings in the present.

7.2.1 Two Schemas of Love: Romantic and Real

In the introduction to the German edition of the first volume of his *Écrits*, Lacan writes that transference is based on love; "a feeling that takes on such a new form in analysis not [that it is any] less illusory but that it gives itself a partner who has a chance to respond, which is not the case in other forms" (1975, 16). Transference positions the Analyst as a respondent to the demand for love, whose presence has the effect of returning to the analysand his or her message in a particular way. In this section, I propose two schematizations of love to explore the way the Analyst responds to the analysand's demand. The first, which I qualify as "romantic" love, allows us to approach the erotic dimension of transference from the initial perspective of an affective encounter. The second, which I refer to as "Real" love, describes the transference relation as the site of the formation of an ethical experience for both parties involved. To this end, I provide an account of how the Analyst aims at an encounter with the register of the Real.

In Seminar VIII (1960–1961), Lacan states that transference "manifests itself in a relationship with someone who speaks" and can thus be understood to sustain the action of speaking itself (*SVIII* 175). Speech is no other than a demand; it presupposes an Other to whom it is addressed and whose signifiers it takes over in its unique formulation. Alan Sheridan notes that what comes from the Other is treated "not so much as a satisfaction of a need, but a response to an appeal, a gift, a token of love" (2001, viii).[1] Sheridan's comments point to the link Lacan establishes between the conceptual triad of need (*besoin*), demand (*demande*) and desire (*désir*). The biological needs of the speaking subject inevitably pass through the defiles of the demand. In analysis the subject who speaks is positioned, as Lacan insists, in both "beyond and shy of demand" (*SVIII* 198). The "beyond" is located in the demand *for love* while the "shy of" is what characterizes it as a condition: desire. Lacan situates the latter in the gap that separates need from the demand that conveys it and correlates desire not with an object that might satisfy it, but with the partial object that causes it: <*a*>. Lacan refers to the "agalma" to explain that the

[1] Sheridan's commentary can be found in the translator's note of *Écrits*: A Selection.

analysand sees his or her object of desire in the Analyst who occupies the position of <*a*>.

Analysis attempts to bring to light the manifestations of the analysand's desire as linked and conditioned by the fantasy that constitutes the transference relation. The analyst plays a transferential role "to the degree to which he is for the analysand what he is not at the level of reality" (*SVIII* 314). Alongside the transfer of speech, imaginary transference involves the projection of images in which the speaking subject expresses or exteriorizes an identifying *imago* onto the analyst's own person. In "Aggressivity in Psychoanalysis" (1948) Lacan writes that the analyst offers the analysand "the pure mirror of an unruffled surface" and must limit oneself to the activity of returning to the analysand his or her own egoic reflection (*ÉS* 12). The analyst must recognize that all demands are demands are to be loved with related the understanding that desire is what lies behind the demand. In the context of analytic experience, Lacan teaches that desire is neither "the appetite for satisfaction, nor the demand for love but the difference that results from the subtraction of the first from the second" (219).

In his early writings, Lacan conceives of love as a function that is based on a fundamentally narcissistic structure: the desire to be desired. Drawing on Freud's distinction between "ego ideal" (*ich-ideal*) and "ideal ego" in Seminar VIII, Lacan defines love in terms of a narcissistic relationship of the subject. At work within the experience of falling in love is the recognition of the substance that forms of the ideal ego. In *(Per)versions of Love and Hate*, Renata Salecl states that "for romantic love to emerge, the real person need not be present; what is necessary is the existence of the image" (1998, 13). Romantic love, in this sense, refers to the way the subject positions the object of their love in the place of the ideal ego. The subject loves this object because of the perfection the subject has striven to reach of his or her own ego. Salecl claims that in romantic love the subject simultaneously "posits the object of his or her love in the place of the ego ideal" (13). When placed in the position of the ego ideal, the love object enables one to perceive oneself in a new and desirable way (e.g., beautiful, loveable, decent).

Romantic love is deceptive because the subject who demands to be loved or who imagines that s/he gives love fails to recognize the desire that is operating within the hollow of a demand for love. By taking the whole person as his or her libidinal object, the subject's perception of love conceals the fact that s/he actually became attracted to the <*a*>; the partial object that causes desire. At the same time, the lover loves in order that the other will see him or her how s/he wants to be seen. Discussing the narcissistic field, Lacan states that "the whole question is to discover how the love object may fulfil a role analogous to the object of desire" (*SXI* 186). Lacan maintains that what we often call love is ignorance; it is also hate. Seen in this way, the object is both something that one admires as well as something that provokes aggression. Paradoxically, the subject destroys what s/he loves most, or as Lacan puts it: "because I love in you something more than you—the object petit a—I destroy you" (*SXI* 263).

The notion of "romantic love" can help draw out Lacan's emphasis that desire is what lies behind the demand for love. The subject's demand is aimed at the Other. Desire for the Other to serve as the support for one's self-image is then projected as a demand placed on actual others. Seen from this angle, Lacan explains that the demand "annuls the particularity of everything that can be granted by transmuting it into a proof of love, and the very satisfactions it obtains for need are reduced to the level of being no more than the crushing of the demand for love" (*ÉS* 219). This results in a situation that is fundamentally unethical. To the extent that "love", in this sense, expresses the narcissistic aim of making one of two or fusing two into one, the destruction of the love object can be seen as the annihilation of subjective difference. Grace Tarpey asserts that romantic love is better understood as a mirage that fills out the void or makes up for the lack of the impossibility of the relationship between the sexes.[2]

In Seminar VIII, Lacan draws on Plato's *Symposium* to thematize the nature of erotic desire from a psychoanalytic point of view. With the bond of love between Socrates and Alcibiades as a focal point, Lacan's seminar shows that, more than a desire for bodies, "eros" is a desire for knowledge. Moreover, Lacan casts the love relationship in opposition to

---

[2] See Grace Tarpey's article, "Lacan's Psychoanalytic Way of Love", *PsychoanalysisLacan*, 1. Available at: https://lacancircle.com.au/psychoanalysislacan-volume-1/. [Accessed 22 April 2021.]

traditional ideologies that see it as a paradigm for that which unites two lovers in reciprocity, complementarity, or fusion. Love in the *Symposium* emphasizes rather the asymmetry and disparity that exists between two parties, not unlike the bond between analyst and analysand. To demonstrate how the erotic relationship generates positions that are not only distinct but unequal, Lacan employs the Greek terms *erastés* (lover) and *erómenos* (beloved). The lover, *erastés*, is the desiring subject; the object s/he lacks characterizes all those who come into contact with him or her. The beloved, *erómenos*, knows not what s/he has and that is what makes him or her so appealing. For Lacan, the two terms that constitute the lover and the beloved do not coincide: "what the one is missing is [not] hidden in the other" (*SVIII* 40).

Although Socrates and Alcibiades are linked by an erotic strength, they do not form a couple. Bruno Moroncini astutely remarks that their relationship is characterized not by good chance but by a bad (or, rather missed) encounter: "when Socrates looks for Alcibiades the latter escapes and when Alcibiades is after Socrates this time it is he who remains impassive" (2009).[3] To clarify the nature of the erotic bond, Lacan insists that "love as a signifier, [...] is a metaphor" (*SVIII* 40). The principle of metaphorical substitution, as discussed previously, is linked to the production of meaning.[4] In analysis, the hysteric traditionally masks desire in symptoms whose meaning s/he cannot say and asks the doctor to give her that meaning or produce knowledge about the desire or eros that possesses her. Similarly, Alcibiades presses Socrates for the signification of his desire; he is someone who desires but remains ignorant as to what he wants. A possible reading of Lacan's *Symposium* as a quasi-prototype of the analytic relationship lies in the fact that love is due to a passion to know that verges on ignorance.

This perspective can also shed light on how love in transference is addressed to the one who we think knows our real truth. Put in slightly different terms, the Discourse of the Analyst occupies an imaginary position of mastery. The Analyst functions as the supposed subject of

[3] See Bruno Moroncini's article, "On Love: Jacques Lacan and Plato's Symposium", *European Journal of Psychoanalysis*. Available at: https://www.journal-psychoanalysis.eu/category/ejp/number-5-6-2016-1-2-ejp/lacan-and-platos-synposium-b-moroncini/. [Accessed 7 February 2021.]

[4] See Chapter 4 "The Point de Capiton: A Story of Two Kants".

knowledge because the analysand posits the Analyst as the Master who can deliver the truth of his or her desire. Lacan explains that "as soon as the subject supposed to know exists somewhere [...] there is transference" (*SXI* 232). However, while the Analyst may have knowledge on his or her side, Lacan insists that s/he must refuse the position of the Master. In this way, the Analyst plays a role similar to that of Socrates who claims to have no knowledge of anything except love. Despite assigning it a central place in ethics, Lacan insists that psychoanalysis must remain just as blind as the love to which it gives rise. In its principled refusal of any supposition of knowledge, psychoanalysis would be a form of love that offers relief from the confidence of all those discourses, past and still to come, that claim to know.

This form of love is perhaps reflected by Socrates who, as Lacan observes, "refuses to enter the scale of the desirable" (*SVIII* 161). Put in the position of beloved, Socrates does not know what he has in him that others could find desirable and refuses to believe that there is anything loveable about him. Even though Alcibiades sees in him the "agalma", Socrates cannot condescend to be the love object. In his commentary on Lacan's Seminar VIII, Bruce Fink claims that "Socrates is presented to us a lover who has never gone through the metaphor of love"; he loves without wishing to be loved or being able to accept love in return (*SVIII* 198). The only position Socrates is willing to occupy is that of the lover, the *erastés*. This means, as Fink suggests, that "although Socrates regularly turns his beloveds into lovers, into men who begin to love him and the knowledge they suppose he has, he himself can never undergo the metaphor of love" (198). Like the working analyst, Socrates understands that despite having been put in the position of beloved, he does not occupy this position at the level of reality.

Fink's comments provide a useful segue into the second schema of love. For Lacan, psychoanalysis introduces a peculiar ethical difficulty: it can no longer base itself on an idealizing view of love as it has been traditionally understood. The bond between doctor and patient, writes John Rajchman, is "unlike that of ancient philosophical *philoi*, and unlike that of Christian [*agape*]"; analysis is neither wisdom nor altruism, and "an analyst is not a good Samaritan" (1991, 19). Lacan insists on the desire of the analyst to guide the analysis. In Seminar XI, Lacan describes the

Analyst's desire as the "desire to obtain an absolute difference" (*SXI* 276). The difference in question sacrifices the imaginary and symbolic features of the love object, allowing the other to be different from oneself. Beyond the narcissistic relationship toward the love object, Lacan's later work stresses the need to encounter the Real, the traumatic object in the subject. I propose to read this as "Real love".

Lacan describes the Analyst's desire as "a desire which intervenes when, confronted with the primary signifier, the subject is in a position to subject himself to it" (*SXI* 276). Offering clarification, Russell Grigg distinguishes between "the analyst as a flesh and blood person and the analyst as a signifier, a place within the transference relation" (2008, 56). The Analyst creates a way of proceeding from his or her own desire in order to be rejected as a master signifier and finally mourned by the subject. This occurs through the de-idealization of the Analyst as a subject supposed to know. By remaining an enigmatic "x" for the analysand, the silence of the Analyst suspends the field of meaning and the symbolic order. The absence of the position of mastery, is perhaps one way that psychoanalysis articulates the void of the Real. The ethical disposition of the Analyst comprises his or her desire to give nothing of what s/he has but to orient the transference as a love aimed at the Real. Since the Real cannot be known as such, the Analyst creates an ethical experience for the analysand to empty words of their meaning and to change his or her relationship to knowledge; to signify the Real differently. For Lacan, this occurs when "the signification of love is produced" in transference, that is, by the poetic substitution of the beloved for the lover (*SVIII* 40).

7.2.2 Two Erotic Domains: Care and Psychagogy

The domain of "erotics" structures Foucault's journey to ancient Greece in the 1980s; it functions as a key reference for a genealogy of ethics and for the changes that occurred in ethical self-constitution between the Classical era and late Antiquity. Along with dietetics and economics, "erotics" figured in the tripartite division that provided the structure of Foucault's plan in *The Use of Pleasure* (1984) and *The Care of the Self* (1984), the second and third volumes of the *History of Sexuality*. In these books, Foucault reads Greek, Hellenistic, and Roman philosophy in terms of the moral problematization of pleasure. In his study of sexual ethics, Foucault employs the term "erotics" to designate problematic relations combining pleasure and power between two unequal parties. This is evident in the practice of erotic relations between adult and adolescent males which gave rise to concern, anxiety, and ethical reflection for the Greeks. Foucault thus situates "erotics" as a field of practical action within which the self appears and which is constituted by its possibilities for success and error, its dangers, its techniques, and tactics for safety, as well as its rewards (McGushin 2007).

In his lectures at the Collège de France between 1982 and 1984, Foucault's finds himself concerned with ancient philosophy, as such, independently of the question of sexual ethics. This is not to suggest that the domain of erotics disappears from Foucault's reflection; rather, it acquires a new problematic. Commentators remark that at play in Foucault's interpretation of ancient philosophical texts is the problematization of his own present (Rajchman 1991; Davidson 2005). Timothy O'Leary attributes Foucault's interest in ancient Greece to an age when "individuals were not tied to their forms of identity by the 'tightest bonds' of power/knowledge apparatuses; but were to an extent free to engage in a work of self-constitution whose guiding principles were not interpretive but aesthetic" (2002, 38). In this section, I identify two erotic domains that structure Foucault's problematization of philosophical discourse through reference to his presentation of Plato's Socratic dialogues.

Foucault provides interpretations of a number of works by Plato during his final years at the Collège de France. In the "Hermeneutics of the Subject" (1981–1982), Foucault reads Plato's *Apology* and *Alcibiades* in which he introduces Socrates as a "man of care". In "The Government of Self and Others" (1982–1983) Foucault presents detailed readings of Plato's *Laches*, *Gorgias*, and *Phaedrus* that reveal the role and forms of ethical *parrhesia* in Socratic dialogue. Foucault makes occasional reference to the *Laws* in the same course, and he offers readings of other letters written by Plato. In the *Courage of Truth* (1983–1984) Foucault relies on his previous accounts of each dialogue and the basic themes they develop in order to trace the major lines of divergence in western philosophical practice. In what follows, I focus on Foucault's presentation of two

Socratic dialogues. Beginning with *Alcibiades*, I highlight the transformation of erotics into a practice of care (*epimeleia heauton*). I then turn to Plato's *Gorgias* to underscore the *parrhesiastic* function of philosophical discourse as "psychagogy"; a term that designates an intense affective relationship that is both erotic and pedagogic.

The term "Socratic dialogue" refers to the dialogues written by Plato in his youth which are marked by a familiar context of a certain political and social milieu. According to Foucault, this milieu comprises "the small world of young aristocrats" who, from an early age, are "consumed by the ambition to prevail over others" and to "enter active, authoritarian and triumphant politics" in the Athenian city-state (*HoS* 44). One problem that arises in this context is whether the authority initially conferred on the male elite by birth, wealth, and membership to the aristocratic world (as was the case of Alcibiades), also gives them the political ability to govern properly. The subject of *Alcibiades I* is an encounter in which Socrates, a penniless sage, convinces the young Alcibiades, heir to one the most prestigious Athenian families, that in order to undertake a successful political career, he must first of all begin to take *care* of himself. For Foucault, the dialogue provides a point of departure and a program for Platonic philosophy in which the Socratic injunction to *care* appears as its first principle. To examine the reasons why Socrates and Alcibiades are brought to the notion of taking *care* of oneself, Foucault considers the dialectic between political and erotic discourse.

In *Technologies of the Self*, Foucault remarks that "an ambivalence is evident in Alcibiades political and erotic vocabulary" (*TS* 23–24). During his adolescence, Alcibiades had many admirers whom he rejected in the bloom of his beauty since he did not wish to be dominated by them. Now that Alcibiades is about to embark on his public and political life in which he will dominate others, his lovers have disappeared. At this point, Socrates intervenes and declares his love for Alcibiades. Socrates will make Alcibiades submit to him in a particular way. In order to be capable of governing others, Alcibiades must first be governed, that is, he must submit to Socrates, his lover, with the aim of strengthening his own will and making it adequate to the tasks of political life. By the same token, Foucault observes that Alcibiades can no longer remain a beloved; "he must become active in the political *and* the love game" (23). The two therefore make a pact in which Alcibiades will undertake practices to ensure his transition in both politics and love. For Foucault, at the intersection of Alcibiades' political ambition and Socrates' philosophical love is the *care of the self* (*epimeleia heauton*) (24).

The Socratic interrogation that follows once the pact has been made brings to light not only Alcibiades' ignorance of what it means to rule effectively, but also the way erotic relationships were structured in Athens. Foucault argues in the "Hermeneutics of the Subject" that the requirement of *care* is thematized as a response to the academic and erotic limits of Athenian pedagogy in which adult men would abandon their pursuit of free-born boys precisely at the moment when they needed a guide in order to actualize the proper *ethos* for political life. Edward McGushin explains that the erotic field was used "as an opportunity for one individual, the lover, experienced as a principle of pleasure and a will to power, to persuade, manipulate, and seduce the other, the beloved, who was at a great disadvantage in the erotic game" (2007, 73). Socrates' task was to compensate for the defective pedagogy which threatened Alcibiades' future by restoring philosophical love to its ethical function. As a new kind of lover who cared for the soul of the beloved, Socrates displaced the erotic relationship from its former situation as a struggle for power in the form of conquest and seduction to a pact between the philosopher, who practices *care*, and the disciple who must learn to free himself of his current way of being.

With the Platonic-Socratic tradition as a focal point, Foucault demonstrates that erotics is transformed into a practice of *care*. The principle of *care* takes on a specific meaning in the context of the "Hermeneutics of the Subject" where Foucault makes use of it to unsettle a dominant way of reading the history of ancient philosophy through the formula of the Delphic injunction "know yourself" (*gnothi seauton*). The latter precept, insists Foucault, should be interpreted "as one of the forms, one of the consequences, as a sort of concrete, precise, and particular application of the general rule": you must take *care* of yourself (*HoS* 5). In *epimeleia*, one performs various exercises, or one engages in a variety of practices which have the deliberate goal of cultivating a certain relationship to the self. This is evident in *Alcibiades I* where the practice of *caring for oneself* in the form of contemplation is intended to resist prevailing forms of the neglect of the self. It also serves to purify Alcibiades' will which has been corrupted by the general opinion and inscribed in his soul as his very identity through an inadequate erotic relationship. In Plato's dialogue, the principle "know yourself" is given a special inflection among the activities of which *care* is composed, as Timothy O'Leary puts it:

> *Alcibiades 1* answers the [...] question—'what is the relation between care of the self and knowledge of the self?'—by suggesting that the knowledge which is a necessary element of the care of the self can only be achieved in and through an 'erotic' attachment between a disciple and a master. It is Socrates's great love for Alcibiades which—even in its purified, 'platonic' form—is the driving force behind bringing Alcibiades to virtue and temperance. (2002, 48)

The relation between *epimeleia heauton* and *gnothi seauton* acquires an even greater significance in the analytic framework of the "Hermeneutics of the Subject" in which Foucault traces "the historically and philosophically modifiable connection between the subject and truth" (*HoS* xxi). This is also one of the rare occasions that Foucault speaks directly and admiringly of Lacan, insisting that he has been "the only psychoanalyst since Freud who has sought to refocus the question of psychoanalysis [...] on the relations between the subject and truth" (30). Crucially, Foucault's comments suggest that Lacan does not subscribe to the Western tradition of "the analytics of truth" which is concerned with how we arrive at and evaluate truths; he engages rather in another type of critical attitude toward truth, less preeminent than the first. According to Foucault "Lacan reintroduces into psychoanalysis the oldest tradition, the oldest questioning, and the oldest disquiet of the *epimeleia heauton*, which was the most general form of spirituality" (30). Here, the question is not so much what *is* true as what it means to us and the societies in which we find ourselves to *say* what is true—the consequences, the risks, in a word, the "costs" of doing so. In this way, Foucault begins his 1982 course with the historical claim that, throughout Antiquity, in different modalities:

> The philosophical question of "how to have access to the truth" and the practice of spirituality (of the necessary transformations in the very being of the subject which will allow access to the truth), these two questions, these two themes, were never separate. (17)

In more succinct terms, Foucault argues that, in Antique spirituality:

> I think we can say that in and of itself an act of knowledge could never give access to the truth unless it was prepared, accompanied, doubled, and completed by a certain transformation of the subject; not of the individual, but of the subject himself in his being as subject. (16)[5]

Erotics, as presented in the Platonic-Socratic tradition (and perhaps, too, in Lacanian analysis), establishes a field in which to locate this spiritual function insofar as it aims to transform the beloved from being an *object* of love into a *subject* who must take up an active relationship to oneself. In addition to the *care of the self*, the problem of the "costs" of truth-telling was raised in Greek Antiquity by the activities of *parrhesia* which introduced a new verbal ethic. Foucault insists that the aim of *parrhesia* is "not to keep the person to whom one speaks dependent on the one who speaks", as in flattery (*HoS* 379). The objective of *parrhesia* is to speak to the other in such a manner that "he will be able to form an autonomous, independent, full and satisfying relationship to himself" (379). Defined as "anti-flattery", Foucault associates *parrhesia* with acting in such a way so that the person to whom one is speaking can find themselves in a situation where they can "leave the relationship with the other person" (379). Exiting the *parrhesiastic* relationship depends on internalizing and subjectivizing a true discourse: "truth, in passing from one to the other in *parrhesia*, seals, ensures, and guarantees the autonomy of the person who received the speech from the person who uttered it" (379).

Another place in which Foucault examines the "pact" between the speaker and the listener is Plato's *Gorgias* where the notion of *parrhesia*

[5] Foucault's comments foreshadow the distinction made in "The Government of Self and Others" (1982–1983) between two Kantian traditions: a formal inquiry of the conditions in which we can have access to truth, and a radical (or "spiritual) inquiry into the practice we must undertake to transform ourselves to have access to truth. See Chapter 4 "*Le Point de Capiton*: A Story of Two Kants".

appears in the philosophical practice of the conduction of individual souls, that is, in the context of "ancient spiritual direction" (*GSO* 367). Focusing on the second half of the dialogue, Foucault devotes significant attention to the exchange that takes place between Socrates and Callicles. Like Alcibiades, Callicles is an Athenian aristocrat with political ambitions to prevail over others. The resistance Callicles encounters differs from that of Alcibiades in that it concerns the Athenian law (*nomos*) of equality which aims to give the same status to everyone. Faced with a predicament in which the advantages of wealth and privilege no longer place him among the upper echelons of the social order, Callicles resorts to other means to acquire his authority. Foucault describes Callicles as a young man who wants to play "the traditional agonistic game in a system which has become egalitarian" (369). Rhetoric, according to Foucault, is the instrument that will enable Callicles to assert his superiority and to restore inequality to "a society on which an attempt to impose an egalitarian structure has been pursued through democratic laws" (369).

At this point in the dialogue Socrates intervenes and proposes an entirely different discursive game which frames the transition from rhetoric to philosophical *parrhesia*. Unlike the *parrhesia*, rhetoric implies no identification of the speaker with what is said. On the contrary, the rhetor strives to establish a bond of force between what is said and the one who is addressed. Rhetoric is a technique of speaking that enables one to persuade others to believe in statements that may or may not be true, that the speaker may or may not believe. In rhetoric there is a *difference* between the speaker and what is said, but an *identity* between the listener and what is said (McGushin 2007). This identity is a desired effect of rhetoric insofar as it places the listener under the power of the speaker. Foucault claims that, for Callicles, rhetoric is a discourse that has only one use: "it is a matter of prevailing over others" (2010, 370). To this, Socrates responds by proposing, in place of Callicles' agonistic game, a test relationship between two souls based on a "natural affinity" (370). Here, Foucault argues that Socratic *parrhesia* establishes a bond between the master and the disciple through which the *tekhne* specific to philosophical discourse "can act on the soul of the other and lead it to truth" (373).

In *Tragedy and Enlightenment* Christopher Rocco claims that the subject of the *Gorgias* is the relationship "between power and morality"; alongside arguments about rhetoric, it portrays a struggle over "who will set the terms of the discourse, and so control both the dialogue and what counts as 'moral in it'" (1997, 76). The struggle between Socrates, the philosopher who sets the formal parameters of the dialogue, and Callicles, the politician who refuses to submit, describes a situation in which there is no final closure. Socrates falls short of convincing Callicles to change his life as well as his beliefs, yet Callicles is unable to sever the tenuous bond that holds them together. After multiple lapses into silence, Callicles re-joins the conversation and admits to being at once attracted to and repelled by Socrates. Their ongoing exchange manifests a dialogue about dialogue, speeches that contain speech, and pauses which reflect on the grounds of its own possibility. Plato's *Gorgias* reveals, among other things, the contested and contestable ground of philosophy and politics; it conveys knowledge of that contestability and the work implied by it. In Rocco's account, *Gorgias* shows us that a pure Socratic dialogue is not always possible because it is conditioned by "the structural, material, and existential realities of power that disable the mutually beneficial search for truth" (78).

Rocco's interpretation of the dialogue between Socrates and Callicles, while helpful, does not account for the significance that Foucault attributes to it in "The Government of Self and Others". Foucault's main interest in Plato's *Gorgias* is to highlight the relationship of the parrhesiastic philosophy to "psychagogy" or the guidance, conduction, and test of the soul. In its psychagogic activity, *parrhesiastic* philosophy addresses itself to "the disciple, the other soul, the person one pursues" (*GSO* 353). In this way, Foucault describes a relationship of "inclusion, reciprocity and twinning" that brings together "pedagogy and erotics" (353). The bond between master and disciple is defined by relations of intense *philia* rather than profound *eros*. Foucault explains that, in order to formulate the test of the truth, the two interlocutors must have "a feeling of benevolence for each other that comes from friendship" (372). Contrasted with the Periclean model of political *parrhesia* in which the use of rhetoric enables one to prevail over others by binding them together in the unity of the command, psychagogy binds two others in the unity of knowledge. Through his notion of *parrhesia*, Foucault endeavors to show that philosophy is not simply a form of knowledge but a style of discourse which aims at the transformation of the subject who speaks and the subject who listens.

7.3 The Ethics of Eros

In this section, I discuss the attempts that Lacan and Foucault make to re-think eros while reflecting on the way in which the eros of their thought can be linked to ethics. I frame this discussion through the lens of an encounter with the work of each thinker and the subjective experience of writing this book. In Sect. 7.3.1 "Foucault: An Erotic Method" I identify the "etho-poetic" aim of Foucault's genealogy to transform the subject engaged in historical or philosophical thinking. Taking inspiration from Lynne Huffer's *Foucault's Strange Eros* (2020), I read "eros" as a verb that articulates possibilities for something other than discipline, domination, and universal morality. I describe the erotic movement of genealogy as an erosive encounter that gnaws at the continuities of knowing and inhabiting the world. Historicism brings to the fore all the fraught ways we are bound to our time and our *ethos*, yet it holds out the prospect of unbinding ourselves from them in a kind of ethical self-release. I relate this description of the ethics of eros to the writing process itself which intruded, interrupted, and suspended my everyday practices of living. I explain how, by returning to this process year after year, I consented to becoming undone by loosening the fabric of my subjectivity as a writer.

Shifting the focus to the Analyst's discourse, I reflect on Rajchman's claims that Lacan makes the eros of not-knowing a principle of a new kind of thought. In Sect. 7.3.2, "Lacan: The Feminine Knower and Its Discourse" I introduce the question of how to grasp the Discourse of the Analyst and the subject position of (not-)knowing it makes available as being sexualized. Through reference to Jeanne Schroeder's *The Four Lacanian Discourses* and Kirsten Campbell's *Jacques Lacan and Feminist Epistemology*, I develop a perspective of how sexual difference is inscribed in Lacan's matrix of the four discourses. Drawing on Lacan's graph of sexuation in Seminar XX: *Encore* (1972–1973), I present the feminine subject in the position of *non all* which represents both an objection to the phallic signifier and a signification of its limit. I conclude Sect. 7.3 with a reflection on my experience working with the discourses of psychoanalysis that signify in excess of what a phallic regime can capture.

7.3.1 Foucault: An Erotic Method

In this section, I summarize the “etho-poetic” dimension of Foucault’s genealogy in terms of an ethical invitation to philosophical investigation as a practical art that transforms both the speaker and the listener. The objective is to develop a preliminary account of how eros and ethics interact in Foucault’s thought. John Rajchman writes of Foucault that perhaps “in our eros we [are] no longer Greek, no longer Christian, no longer Freudian but [are] becoming something else” (1991, 87). As a starting point, I take this “something else” to be a salient feature of Foucault’s eros which begins and ends as an ethics that does not tell us who we are or what to do but leaves open the space for curiosity and innovation. To this end, I describe Foucault as an erotic thinker through reference to the method and movement of genealogy which does not take the ethics as a given but starts by putting ethical ideals in question.

In an interview conducted by Michael Bess in 1980, Foucault was asked about the moral elements on which he bases ethical action toward others. To this Foucault responds with the goal of offering “refusal, curiosity, and innovation”.[6] He goes on to take aim at moral philosophy specifically: “I think at the heart of this there’s a misunderstanding about the function of philosophy, of the intellectual, of knowledge in general: and that is that it’s up to them to tell us what is good”.[7] Foucault’s statement echoes the Nietzschean rejection of forms of morality that would be acceptable to everyone which he describes as “catastrophic” (1996, 473).[8] In his genealogy of morality, Nietzsche exposed the violence—colonial

---

[6] Michel Foucault, “An Interview with Michel Foucault,” conducted by Michael Bess, November 3, 1980. Available at: https://michaelbess.net/foucault-interview/ [Accessed 31 July 2020].

[7] Ibid.

[8] See Foucault, M. (1996) “The Return of Morality” in Lotringer, S. (ed.) *Foucault Live: Collected Interviews, 1961–1984*, New York, N.Y., Semiotext(e).

conquests, slavery, and genocide—that lie at the bottom of "all good things" (2007, 82). As a method of critique, genealogy submits ethical ideals to the historical contingency of their violent formation in the production of moral conscience. Unlike normative moralities and deontology, genealogy signals a refusal to take ethics at face value; it mobilizes a mode of questioning.

In his text *The Question of Ethics*, Charles Scott argues that genealogy "puts in question the body of values that led to the questioning" (1990, 1). For Foucault, this mode of questioning applies not only to the work of historical analysis but to that of philosophical thought itself. In an interview conducted by Gerard Raulet, Foucault states that the function of the diagnosis of ourselves in the present involves "following lines of fragility" in order to grasp "how that which is might no longer be that which is" (*EST* 449–50). As a mode of self-questioning, genealogy opens the space for "concrete freedom, that is, of possible transformation" (450). Edward McGushin reiterates this view in claiming that Foucault's historicism is "etho-poetic" in that it seeks not to achieve objective historical truth but to transform the subject engaged in historical and philosophical thinking (2007, xxiii). Genealogy takes on a creative dimension through the process of "fictioning", or as Foucault puts it:

> It seems to me that the possibility exists for fiction to function in truth, for a fictional discourse to induce effects of truth, and for bringing it about that a true discourse engenders or "manufactures" something that does not as yet exist, that is, "fictions" it. (*EST* 193)

The activity of "fictioning" follows a double movement. On one hand, the microphysics of power that genealogy brings to light reveal that history, truth and life are made, invented, and fashioned. On the other hand, Foucault insists that inscribed within the work of historical analysis is the implication that "since these things have been made, they can be unmade, so long as we know how it was they were made" (1998, 450). The unmaking that occurs in the archive works against the interiorization of moralities that mask their own violence through a counter movement which "speaks" to the outside.[9] The genealogist creates new fictions whose effects of truth transform the listener in terms that are both epistemic and ethical. The work of manufacturing a fictional truth alters the subject-object relation that defines the encounter between the knower and the known. As a discontinuous movement of contingency, genealogy works by dissolving interiority through repeated gestures in history that leave in suspense anything that might take on the appearance of completion in the present or of rest in truth.

In her recent text *Foucault's Strange Eros*, Lynne Huffer proposes to read "eros" in Foucault as an instance of *ethopoiesis* at work: "eros as a verb, out of sync with the present, returning us as strange" (2020, 46). Eros mimics the erosive grammar of genealogy as a paradoxical doing and undoing; it implies "an embodied thinking, a feeling praxis" that can shake up the present through a process of distancing, dispersing, and effacing (64). As a preverbal verb that names a conditioning "can-do-ness", Huffer argues that eros signals concrete practices of freedom "that cohere and dissolve not sequentially but simultaneously" (25). Eros is a verb that frees not by providing a system or field with its own codes and knowledges but by articulating possibilities for something other than discipline, domination, and universal morality (25). At work in eros is the recognition of the ethical and political implications of genealogy as a fight for de-institutionalizing and de-subjectifying practices. Like the erotic movement of genealogy that exposes meaning-making as the temporary result of sedimentation, Huffer explains that eros unleashed "coils and recoils" through a mode of questioning in which our ways of living, knowing and inhabiting the world appear as both bound and unbound to the mast of time (20).

Huffer's account of "eros undisciplined" overlaps with Foucault's vision of ethics as an experiment in living, an experiment, moreover, that seeks not a transcendent flight into something new but an ethical self-release or subtle self-undoing. As Foucault writes in the *History of Sexuality* vol. 2, his work is motivated by "that which enables one to get free of oneself"

---

[9] In Chap. 2, I presented the epistemology driving Foucault's "hystorical critique", through reference to the Nietzschean analysis of de-implication, as opening genealogy to the "Outside of Knowing", that is, against the interiority of philosophical discourse and the theoretical structure of knowledge-desire-truth in Aristotle.

(*HS2* 8). He goes on to locate "the value of the passion for knowledge" not in the production of "a certain amount of knowledgeableness" but in "knower's straying afield of himself" (8). The action of straying is subtractive; it consists in a deductive dismantling of the self rather than its wholesale negation. Ethical experiments in living are those that target a dissolution of the self, not as substance but a temporally contingent and nested set of connections. For Foucault, the main interest in life and work is to become something other than what we were in the beginning; to become again what we never were. In discussion of "Truth, Power, Self" in 1982, Foucault reiterates this view with the following rhetorical question:

> If you knew when you began a book what you would say at the end, do you think that you would have the courage to write it? What is true for writing and for a love relationship is true also for life. The game is worthwhile insofar as we don't know what will be the end. (*TS* 9)

Foucault's experiments in living suggest a confrontation with a limit that he calls de-subjectivation. Commentators often cite Foucault's forays into drug or sex-induced limit experiences—his LSD trip in Death Valley or his involvement with sadomasochism—as examples of the de-subjectifying practices he has in mind. The reality, is perhaps, more sober and less self-indulgent. As indicated in the passage above, Foucault seeks in his writings to get free of himself. The practice of writing is slow and recursive; a hollowing out of the self over time compared to the explosive experience of losing oneself by getting high or surrendering to the thrall of kinky sex. This is not to suggest that Foucault privileges writing over other kinds of experiments in living; freedom's task is not that of cleaving to principles that tell us how best to live; rather, it involves creating something new and perhaps different that is worthy of being lived. The fact remains that Foucault was an intellectual and wrote books for a living. I insist on this point to convey something of my own experience in writing this book.

Given that I dedicated a portion of research to interpreting Foucault's genealogy through the lens of the Hysteric's Discourse, it makes sense to claim that my experience began as an encounter with the unreason of an erotic method. Alongside what Lynne Huffer calls "Foucault's strange eros", I engaged in a writing process that could equally be described as a strange kind of labor carried out on myself. Like the movement Foucault describes in "The Thought of the Outside" which intrudes on the subject's interiority, "drawing it out of itself", there were days when words seemed to enter me suddenly in a haphazard fashion (1998, 163). Sometimes I would receive with remarkable clarity the concluding remarks of a chapter I had yet to write or the beginning of a problematic that still needed working through. These flashes of insight, although initially captivating, were transient and short lived. To grasp their meaning or non-meaning, significance or insignificance, would require long hours of tedious work. In that process, I used light sparingly only in order to illuminate the gaps in my not-knowing.

My experience of writing engaged with Foucault's erotic method in ways that suspended and transformed my everyday practices of living. In "A Preface to Transgression" Foucault describes not the crossing of a line but a suspension of the relation that gives the line, what he calls the distance that "opens at the heart of the limit" (1998, 74). For Foucault, it is an experiment with limits that brings about an experience of suspension necessary for de-subjectivation. As it relates to my own experiment in limits, writing took the form of both an erosive and recursive movement. The writing frequently meandered; it was endless and crablike. Like a poem it folded over on itself, wandered away for a time, and returned back again intruding and interrupting on my life. With each new version, revision, and edit, there was not only something new on the page but something that was falling or fading away into the background whenever I spoke about it. Through my returns to this process year after year, I consented to coming undone by loosening the knotted fabric of my subjectivity as a writer. I continue this reflection in the following and final section.

7.3.2 Lacan: The Feminine Knower and its Discourse

In his book *Truth and Eros*, John Rajchman asserts that the difficulty of Lacan's teaching and style "refuses the knowledge of a Good or Ideal" and makes "the eros of our not-knowing the principle of a new kind of philosophy" (1991, 26). In this section, I consider Rajchman's comments in terms of the positions of knowing made available by the discourses of psychoanalysis: the Hysteric and the Analyst. In Seminar XVII: *The Other Side of Psychoanalysis* (1969–1970) Lacan demonstrates that all knowledge is based on a signifying articulation which is constituted by a system of differential elements that link one signifier <S1> to another <S2>. Articulated systems of knowledge position the speaking subject at certain points within those systems. For Lacan, the speaking subject also emerges within the field of sexual difference. This provides an occasion to raise the parallel question of how we might understand the four discourses and their corresponding positions of knowing as being sexed. Distinguishing Lacan's thought from other forms, Slavoj Žižek states that:

> [o]ne of the crucial differences between psychoanalysis and philosophy concerns the status of sexual difference: for philosophy the subject is not inherently sexed [...] whereas psychoanalysis promulgates sexualization into a kind of formal, a priori, condition of the very emergence of the subject. (1998, 81)

From the outset of his seminar, Lacan presents each discourse as the inverse of another discourse. The Master is the "other side" of the discourse of psychoanalysis referred to in the title. Although Lacan does not address the issue, implicitly the Discourse of the University is the "other side" of that of the Hysteric. One way of approaching the question of sexual difference is through the lens of the sexual impasse that underlies the inverted relation of discourse in Lacan's theory. In her text *The Four Lacanian Discourses*, Jeanne Schroeder proposes to read Lacan's concept of the sexual non-relationship in terms of the opposition it establishes between the discourses of power, on one side, and the discourses of critique, on the other. From the perspective of the sexual impasse, the terms "feminine" and "masculine" do not refer to persons either biologically or socially identified as male or female. Schroeder maintains that "masculine" and "feminine" refer to incompatible ways of confronting the alienation of the speaking subject in language and the contradiction that inhabits all concepts.

For Schroeder, the "masculine" attitude designates denial; "it attempts to resolve contradiction in order to create a complete and closed social universe" (2008, 1). The masculine position is characterized by the determinability and commensurability of the symbolic order; it says that the law is complete, knowledge has a determinate object, and everything can be measured and placed within an order. By contrast, the "feminine" attitude accepts contradiction and recognizes that rather than being completely bound to the symbolic order, the feminine position partially escapes it. Schroeder describes the feminine position in terms of an insistence on the "incompleteness of the law, the inadequacy of all comparisons, and the slippage of signification" which reveals the lacunae of meaning (127). Schroeder thus explains that the Master and the University are structurally discourses of power and therefore masculine, whereas the Hysteric and the Analyst are structurally discourses of critique and so feminine.

This outline helps illustrate Lacan's claim in Seminar XX: *Encore* (1972–1973) that there is no sexual relationship. That sexuality is an impossibility means that it cannot be bridged in the symbolic order. For Lacan, the two sexes are not complements that can be fitted together to form a whole. When combined, the feminine and masculine positions produce a strange mélange of overlaps and gaps. Lacan intends to underscore that if individuals were able to satisfy each other and join as one, they would lose their subjectivity and individuality. The upshot of Lacan's aphorism is that despite the desire to merge with one another our individuation holds out the possibility for us to achieve something along the lines of "love".

In Seminar XVII, Lacan responds to the question "what is the love of truth" by first situating himself within the Analyst's discourse (*SXVII* 52). For the Analyst, the "love of truth" necessarily implies "the love of weakness" (52). The point Lacan wishes to make is that truth itself is impotent with respect to the whole. The Analyst's love of truth enables the analysand to know this weakness, to recognize the failure and limits of its knowledge. If the Analyst positions him or herself as the One who can intervene in the analysand's knowledge through an act of interpretation that is comprehensive and complete, s/he deprives the subject of the possibility of coming to their own truth. The Analyst must instead institute the subject as the "master" of their speech who must refuse the position of mastery. In her text *Jacques Lacan and Feminist Epistemology* Kirsten Campbell proposes to read Lacan's schema not as "describing the knowledge of the analyst but that of the analysand" (2004, 80). Campbell's reformulation of Lacan's theory retains the concept of the structure of the Discourse of the Analyst but emphasizes the position of the knowing subject which that discourse produces.

Freud's experience with the hysteric subject provides one example of how the analytic discourse describes the analysand's knowledge. In her sexuality, the hysteric represented a defiance to the "mastery" of medicine and to the medical norms of health. Through his encounter with hysteria, Freud confronted the limits of what his medical training had taught him. In the hysteric's symptoms Freud found that one desires something other than one's good for which there is no generalized "normal" manifestation. John Rajchman writes that "the symptoms of the hysteric were not to be defined by the Ideal of a healthy sexuality; it was on the contrary the ideals of health that had to be rethought" in order to come to terms with the hysteric subject and her desire (1991, 24–25). The theoretical question that emerges from this scenario raises the ethical difficulty of what to do about a desire for which there is no cure. While Freud's legacy expressly left aside the question of what women want, Lacan confronts the question in Seminar XX which leads to a reworking of his theory of the female subject.

In this seminar, Lacan introduces his graph of sexuation which, like his earlier accounts of sexed subjectivity, represents sexed identity in relation to the "phallic function". Bruce Fink explains that the phallic function is "the function that institutes lack, that is, the alienating function of language" (1995, 203). The feminine and masculine positions that are represented by Lacan's formulae of sexuation are structured by a relation to the phallus. For this reason, Lacan claims that a relation between the sexes is an impossibility. Lacan holds that the phallic function describes the male subject as being "whole" or "all" (*SXX* 79). Elie Ragland-Sullivan understands the male subject as one who "unconsciously perpetuates the suppression of the person's own division and the belief in her or his autonomy" (1987, 305). In the position of mastery, the masculine subject defines his universality in relation to the Other who lacks the phallus.

The female subject occupies this other position which Lacan writes as: ~~The~~ Woman.

When read from the side of the masculine subject, Lacan's graph of sexuation positions the female subject as an exception to the phallic signifier and thus as a signification of its limit. Lacan argues that "when any speaking being whatsoever situates itself under the banner "women", it is on the basis of the following—that it grounds itself as being not-whole in situating itself in the phallic function" (*SXX* 72). Kirsten Campbell understands the *not all* of the female subject as a failure of the signifier to represent her sexed subjectivity (2004, 88). Seen in this way, the position of the *not all* is not an ontological description of women but a description of the position of the female subject is socio-symbolic relations. The position of the *not all* is an objection to the masculine universal. For Lacan, ~~The~~ Woman is a fantasy which affirms that the masculine subject has the phallus. The bar that crosses through "the" shows that the masculine fantasy of ~~The~~ Woman is an impossibility. Lacan states that the position of the *not all* is not that of negation or contradiction but of "indeterminacy" (*SXX* 103). The phallus fails to effect closure of the symbolic order because there is always something "more".

While it is beyond the scope of the current chapter to explore Lacan's theory of female sexuality, I conclude this section and the book itself with a reflection on my experience working with the discourses of psychoanalysis that signify in excess of what a phallic regime can capture. I preface this discussion with a commentary on Lacan. Despite the authoritative bodies and hierarchies that have been put in place to ensure the procedural transmission of Lacan's teachings, there is a dimension to his thought which opens to a larger audience, and which perhaps cannot be transmitted in the same way. The difficulty—indeed, obscurity—of Lacan's style stems partly from the fact that he was first and foremost an orator whose sayings were recorded and translated into his *Écrits*. In the work I undertook to untangle that difficulty over the past years, I encountered something more than what I knew what to do with.

My entry into Lacan began with his theory of the four discourses which lack any systematized approach. One would certainly be mistaken to look for a linear step-by-step method for discourse analysis in Lacan. His writings are often without fixed rules and rubrics and as such are prone to all sorts of ambiguities. The algebraic terms that make up the discourses condense and embody a substantial quantity of Lacan's theorization, yet each are also highly polyvalent. In my research, I worked gropingly by lingering over the ambiguity of my not-knowing while registering the heuristics made available by it. The ambiguity allowed me to approach Foucault not as an object to be known, but rather as an object of libidinal investment. My lingering became a means for me to follow a blind attraction intuitively, sometimes circuitously, until it led somewhere or simply fizzled out into a dead end. The movement it generated mimicked the notion of eros undisciplined that frees by awakening and releasing my cravings and aversions.

Alongside this libidinal reality, I was tasked with the project of establishing a scholarly work of research. A subject who is after the knowledgeableness of their object can rationally choose a route which suits their tastes whether it be effective, ambitious or simple. A subject who is bound by a libidinal investment takes on the difficulty of oneself and certainly not always by choice since the forces at work seem *plus fort que moi*. It is perhaps worth mentioning that no individual could be exclusively masculine or feminine. Similarly, no subject can speak within only one discourse. Each individual moves from one discourse to another discourse. This book focused primarily on the discourses of psychoanalysis and the feminine positions of knowing they enable. I learned from this experience that rather than being totally bound by the social and symbolic orders, I partially escape them. It is by occupying the feminine position of the *non all* that new knowledges can be invented and read.

References

Campbell, K. (2004) Jacques Lacan and Feminist Epistemology. London: Routledge.

Davidson, A. (2005) "Ethics as Ascetics: Foucault, the History of Ethics, and Ancient Thought", in Gutting, G. (ed.) *The Cambridge Companion to Foucault*. New York: Cambridge University Press, pp. 123–148.

Fink, B. (1995) *The Lacanian Subject between Language and Jouissance*. New Jersey: Princeton University Press.

Foucault, M. (1986). *The Use of Pleasure: The History of Sexuality Vol. II*. New York: Vintage.
Foucault, M.(1988) *Technologies of the Self: A Seminar with Michel Foucault*, Martin, L. H., Gutman, H. & Hutton, P. H. (eds.). London: Tavistock.
Foucault, M. (1996) *Foucault live: Interviews, 1961–1984,* Lotringer, S. (ed). Translated from the French by L. Hochroth, & J. Johnston. New York: Semiotext(e).
Foucault, M. (1997) *Ethics: Subjectivity and Truth*, Paul Rabinow (ed.). Translated from the French by R. Hurley and others. New York: New Press.
Foucault, M. (1998) *Aesthetics, Method, and Epistemology* (*Essential Works of Foucault*, 1954–1984, *Vol. 2*), Faubion, J. D. (ed.). Translated from the French by R. Hurley. New York: The New Press.
Foucault, M. (2005) *The Hermeneutics of the Subject: Lectures at the Collège de France 1981–1982*, Gros, F. (ed.). Translated from the French by G. Burchell. New York: Palgrave Macmillan.
Foucault, M. (2007) *The Politics of Truth*, Lotringer, S. (ed.). Translated from the French by L. Hochroth & C. Porter. Los Angeles: Semiotext(e).
Foucault, M. (2010) *The Government of Self and Others: Lectures at the Collège de France, 1982–1983*, Gros, F. (ed.). Translated from the French by G. Burchell. New York: Palgrave Macmillan.
Grigg, R. (2008) *Lacan, Language, and Philosophy*. New York: SUNY Press.
Huffer, L. (2020) *Foucault's Strange Eros*. New York: Columbia University Press.
Lacan, J. (1975) Introduction à l'édition allemande d'un premier volume des Écrits. *Scilicet*, 5, Paris: Éditions du Seuil.
Lacan, J. (1978) *The Seminar of Jacques Lacan, Book XI: The Four Fundamental Concepts of Psychoanalysis*, J. A. Miller (ed.). Translated from the French by A. Sheridan. New York/London: W. W. Norton & Company.
Lacan, J. (1998*) The Seminar XX, Encore: On Feminine Sexuality, the Limits of Love and Knowledge*, Miller, J. A. (ed.). Translated from the French by B. Fink. New York: W. W. Norton & Company.
Lacan, J. (2001) *Écrits: A Selection.* Translated from the French by A. Sheridan. London: Routledge.
Lacan, J. (2007) *The Seminar of Jacques Lacan, Book XVII: The Other Side of Psychoanalysis, 1969–1970,* Miller, J. A. (ed.). Translated from the French by R. Grigg. New York: W.W. Norton and Company.
Lacan, J. (2015) *The Seminar, Book VIII. Transference*, Miller, J. A. (ed.). Translated from the French by B. Fink. Cambridge: Polity.

Mcgushin, E. (2007) *Foucault's Askesis: An Introduction to the Philosophical Life*. Evanston: Northwestern University Press.

Moroncini, B. (2009) "On Love. Jacques Lacan and Plato's Symposium" *European Journal of Psychoanalysis*, 25. Available at: https://www.journal-psychoanalysis.eu/on-love-jacques-lacan-and-platos-symposium/ [Accessed: 22 January 2022].

O'Leary, T. (2002) *Foucault and the Art of Ethics*. London: Continuum.

Ragland-Sullivan, E. (1987) *Jacques Lacan and the Philosophy of Psychoanalysis*. Urbana/Chicago: University of Illinois Press.

Rajchman, J. (1991) *Truth and Eros: Foucault, Lacan and the Question of Ethics*. New York/London: Routledge.

Rocco, C. (1997) *Tragedy and Enlightenment: Athenian Political Thought and the Dilemmas of Modernity*. Berkeley: University of California Press.

Salecl, R. (1998) *(Per)versions of love and hate*. London: Verso.

Schroeder, J. L. (2008) *The Four Lacanian Discourses: or Turning Law Inside-out*. London: Birbeck Law.

Scott, C. E. (1990) *The Question of Ethics: Nietzsche, Foucault, Heidegger*. Bloomington: Indiana University.

Sheridan, A. (2015) *Michel Foucault: The Will to Truth*. Abingdon, OX: Routledge.

Žižek, S. (1998) "Four Discourses, Four Subjects", in Žižek, S. (ed.) *Cogito and the Unconscious*. Durham: University of Duke Press, pp. 74–113.

Bibliography

Allen, A. (2008) *The Politics of Our Selves: Power, Autonomy, and Gender in Contemporary Critical Theory*. New York: Columbia University Press.

Allouch, J. (2017) *La Psychanalyse est-elle un exercice spirituel?: réponse À Michel Foucault*. Paris: Epel Editions.

Andía, J. R. (2015), *Michel Foucault,* Review *of Foucault's Lectures on the Will to Know*. http://journals.openedition.org/lectures/18113 [Accessed: 20 January 2021].

Barker, P. (1998) *Michel Foucault: An Introduction*. Edinburgh: Edinburgh University Press.

Bernauer, J. (1990) *Michel Foucault's Force of Flight: Toward an Ethics for Thought*. London: Humanities Press.

Bernauer, J., & Rasmussen, D. (1988) *The Final Foucault*. Cambridge: MIT Press.

Borch-Jacobsen, M. (1991) *Lacan: The Absolute Master*. Translated from the French by D. Brick. Stanford: Stanford University Press.

Bou Ali, N., & Goel, R. (2020) *Lacan contra Foucault: Subjectivity, Sex and Politics*. New York: Sydney Bloomsbury Academic.

Bowie, M. (1991) *Lacan*. Cambridge: Harvard University Press.

Bracher, M. (1993) *Lacan, Discourse, and Social Change: A Psychoanalytic Cultural Criticism*. Ithaca: Cornell University Press.

J. L. Davis, *Reading Foucault Through Lacan*, The Palgrave Lacan Series,
https://doi.org/10.1007/978-3-031-69738-8

———. (1994) "On the Psychological and Social Functions of Language: Lacan's Theory of the Four Discourses", in M. Bracher, M. W. Alcorn Jr., R. J. Corthell, & F. Massardier-Kenney (eds.) *Lacanian Theory of Discourse: Subject, Structure and Society*, New York/London: New York University Press.

Braunstein, N. (2003) "Desire and Jouissance in the Teachings of Lacan", in Rabate, J. M. (ed.) *The Cambridge Companion to Lacan*. Cambridge: Cambridge University Press, pp. 102–115.

Breuer, J., & Freud, S. (1974) *Studies on Hysteria*. Harmondsworth: Penguin Books.

Campbell, K. (2004) Jacques Lacan and Feminist Epistemology. London: Routledge.

Canguilhem, G. (1991) *The Normal and the Pathological*. Translated from the French by C. R. Fawcett with R. S. Cohen. New York: Zone Books.

Caputo, J. (2004) "On Not Knowing Who We Are: Madness, Hermeneutics, and the Night of Truth in Michel Foucault", in Bernauer, J. W., & Carrette, J. R. (eds.) *Michel Foucault and Theology: The Politics of Religious Experience*. Aldershot: Ashgate, pp. 117–139.

Carroll, D. (1982) "Disruptive Discourse and Critical Power: The Conditions of Archaeology and Genealogy", *Humanities in Society*, 5 (3–4), pp. 175–200.

Chatelard, D. (2016) "Du bien-dire et du réel dans la psychanalyse ", *Psychanalyse*, 35 (1), pp. 39–45.

Copjec, J. (1994) *Read My Desire: Lacan Against the Historicists*. London: Verso.

Cottet, S. (2012) *Freud and the Desire of the Psychoanalyst*. London: Karnac.

Darriba, V., & D'escragnolle, M. (2017) "The Presence of Capitalism in Lacan's Theory of Discourse", *Ágora: Estudos em Teoria Psicanalítica*, 20 (2), pp. 543–558. Available at: https://doi.org/10.1590/1809-44142017002012 [Accessed: 12 February 2020].

David-Ménard, M. (1989) *Hysteria from Freud to Lacan: Body and Language in Psychoanalysis*. Ithaca, New York: Cornell University Press.

———. (2010) "About Anti-Oedipus". *Recherches en psychanalyse*, 10, pp. 202–212. Available at https://doi.org/10.3917/rep.010.0021 [Accessed 6 October 2019].

Davidson, A. (2005) "Ethics as Ascetics: Foucault, the History of Ethics, and Ancient Thought", in Gutting, G. (ed.) *The Cambridge Companion to Foucault*. New York: Cambridge University Press, pp. 123–148.

De Kesel, M. (2009) *Eros and Ethics: Reading Jacques Lacan's Seminar VII*. Albany: SUNY Press.

De Saussure, F. (1959) *Course in General Linguistics*. Translated from the French by W. Baskin, Bailly C., & Sechehaye, A. (eds.). New York: Philosophical Library.

Deleuze, G., Guattari, F. (1983) *Anti-Oedipus: Capitalism and Schizophrenia*. Translated from the French by R. Hurley, M. Seem, H. R. Lane. Minneapolis: University of Minnesota Press.

Derrida, J. (1982) *Of Grammatology*. Translated from the French by G. Spivak. Baltimore: John Hopkins University Press.

Dolan, F. M. (1993) "The Philosophical Laughter of Michel Foucault", *Qui Parle,* 6 (2), pp. 131–149. Available at: http://www.jstor.org/stable/20685979 [Accessed: 27 January 2020].

Dolar, M. (2006) Hegel as the Other Side of Psychoanalysis, in Grigg, R., & Clemens, J. (eds.) *Jacques Lacan and the Other Side of Psychoanalysis: Reflections on Seminar XVII*. Durham: Duke University Press, pp. 129–154.

Dreyfus, H., & Rabinow, P. (1982) *Michel Foucault: Beyond Structuralism and Hermeneutics*. London: Routledge.

Dumézil, G. (1941) *Jupiter, Mars, Quirinus: Essai sur la Conception Indo-Européenne de la Société et sur les Origines de Rome*. Paris : Gallimard.

———. (1968) *Mythe et Epopée, vol. 1: L'Idéologie des Trois Fonctions dans les Epopées des Peuples Indo-Européens*. Paris: Gallimard.

Elden, S. (2017) *Foucault the birth of power*. Malden: MA Polity Press.

———. (*2008*) "*Strategies for waging peace*: *Foucault* as a *collaborateur*", in Dillon, M., & Neal, A. (eds.), *Foucault on Politics, Security and War*. London: Palgrave, pp. 21–39.

Eribon, D. (1991) *Michel Foucault*. Translated from the French by B. Wing. Cambridge: Harvard University Press.

Evangelou, A. (2017) *Philosophizing Madness from Nietzsche to Derrida*. Cham, Switzerland: Palgrave Macmillan.

Evans, D. (1996) *An Introductory Dictionary of Lacanian Psychoanalysis*. New York/London: Routledge.

Eyers, T. (2012) *Lacan and the Concept of the "Real"*. Basingstoke: Palgrave Macmillan.

Feldman, A. J. (2019) "Philosophy and Social Criticism Power, Labour Power and Productive Force in Foucault's Reading of Capital", *Philosophy and Social Criticism*, 45 (3), pp. 307–333.

Fink, B. (1995) *The Lacanian Subject between Language and Jouissance*. New Jersey: Princeton University Press.

———. (1998) "The Master Signifier and the Four Discourses", in Nobus, D., (ed.) *Key Concepts of Lacanian Psychoanalysis*. London: Rebus.

———. (1999) *A Clinical Introduction to Lacanian Psychoanalysis: Theory and Technique*. Massachusetts: Harvard University Press.

———.(2015) *Lacan on Love: An Exploration of Lacan's Seminar VIII, Transference*. Cambridge: Polity Press.

Flynn, T. (1985) "Truth and Subjectivation in the Later Foucault", *Journal of Philosophy*, 82 (10), pp. 531–540.

Forrester, J. (1990) *The Seductions of Psychoanalysis: Freud, Lacan, and Derrida*. Cambridge: Cambridge University Press.

Foucault, M. (1976) *Mental Illness and Psychology*. Translated from the French by A. Sheridan. New York: Harper and Row.

———. (1977) "Nietzsche, Genealogy, History", in Bouchard, D. F. (ed.) *Language, Counter-memory, Practice: Selected Essays and Interviews*. Ithaca, NY: Cornell University Press, pp. 139–164.

———. (1980a) *Power/Knowledge: Selected Interviews and Other Writings 1972–1977*. New York: Pantheon.

———. (1980b) "An Interview with Michel Foucault," conducted by M. Bess, November 3, 1980. Available at: https://michaelbess.net/foucault-interview [Accessed: 31 July 2020].

———. (1981) "The Order of Discourse", in Young, R. (ed.) *Untying the Text: A Post-Structuralist Reader*. London: Routledge, pp. 48–78.

———. (1982) "The Subject and Power", *Critical Inquiry*, 8(4), pp. 777–795. Available at: http://www.jstor.org/stable/1343197 [Accessed: 27 January 2021]

———. (1982c) *The Archaeology of Knowledge: and the Discourse on Language*. Translated from the French by A. Sheridan. New York: Vintage Books.

———. (1986) "A Preface to Transgression", in Bouchard, F. & Simon, S. (eds.) *Language, Counter-Memory, Practice: Selected Essays and Interviews*. New York: Cornell University Press. (1977b, pp. 29–52).

———.(1988a) *The History of Sexuality, Volume 3: The Care of the Self.* Translated from the French by R. Hurley. New York: Vintage Books.

———. (1988b) *Madness and Civilization: A History of Insanity in the Age of Reason*. Translated from the French by R. Howard. New York: Vintage Books.

———.(1988c) *Technologies of the Self: A Seminar with Michel Foucault*, Martin, L. H., Gutman, H. & Hutton, P. H. (eds.). London: Tavistock.

———. (1990a) *Politics, Philosophy, Culture Interviews and Other Writings 1977–1984*. Kritzman, L. D. (ed). New York: Routledge.

———. (1990b) *The History of Sexuality, Volume 1: An Introduction*. Translated from the French by R. Hurley. New York: Vintage Books.
———. (1990c) *The History of Sexuality, Volume 2: The Use of Pleasure*. Translated from the French by R. Hurley. New York: Vintage Books.
———. (1991) *Remarks on Marx: Conversations with Duccio Trombadori*. Translated from the French by R. J. Goldstein, & J. Cascaito. New York: Semiotext(e).
———. (1994a) *The Order of Things: An Archaeology of the Human Sciences*. Translated from the French by A. Sheridan. New York: Vintage Books.
———. (1994b) *Dits et écrits, 1954–1969*, vol. 1. Paris: Gallimard.
———. (1994c) *Dits et écrits 1954–1988*, vol. IV. ed. Paris: Gallimard.
———. (1995) *Discipline and Punish: The Birth of the Prison*. Translated from the French by A. Sheridan. New York: Vintage Books.
———. (1996) *Foucault live: Interviews, 1961–1984,* Lotringer, S. (ed). Translated from the French by L. Hochroth, & J. Johnston. New York: Semiotext(e).
———. (1997) *Ethics: Subjectivity and Truth*, Paul Rabinow (ed.). Translated from the French by R. Hurley and others. New York: New Press.
———. (1998) *Aesthetics, Method, and Epistemology* (*Essential Works of Foucault,* 1954–1984, *Vol. 2*), Faubion, J. D. (ed.). Translated from the French by R. Hurley. New York: The New Press.
———. (2000) "Truth and Juridical Forms", in Faubion, J. (ed.) *Foucault: Power*. New York: New Press. pp. 31–35.
———. (2001) *Fearless Speech*, Pearson, J. (ed.). Translated from the French by J. Pearson. Los Angeles: Semiotext(e).
———. (2003) *Society Must Be Defended: Lectures at the Collège de France 1975–1976,* Bertani, M., & Fontana, A. (eds.). Translated from the French by D. Macey. New York: Picador.
———. (2005) *The Hermeneutics of the Subject: Lectures at the Collège de France 1981–1982*, Gros, F. (ed.). Translated from the French by G. Burchell. New York: Palgrave Macmillan.
———. (2007) *The Politics of Truth*, Lotringer, S. (ed.). Translated from the French by L. Hochroth & C. Porter. Los Angeles: Semiotext(e).
———. (2008a) *Psychiatric Power: Lectures at the Collège de France, 1973–1974*, Lagrange, J. (ed.). Translated from the French by G. Burchell. New York: Picador.
———. (2008b) *Introduction to Kant's Anthropology*, Nigro, R. (ed.). Los Angeles: Semiotext(e).

———. (2010a) *The Government of Self and Others: Lectures at the Collège de France, 1982–1983*, Gros, F. (ed.). Translated from the French by G. Burchell. New York: Palgrave Macmillan.

———. (2010b) *The Birth of Biopolitics: Lectures at the Collège de France, 1978–1979*, Senellart, M. (ed.). Translated from the French by G. Burchell. New York: Palgrave Macmillan.

———.. (2010c) *History of Madness*. Translated from the French by J. Murphy and J. Khalfa. Oxon: Routledge.

———.. (2011) *The Courage of Truth (the Government of Self and Others II): Lectures at the Collège de France, 1983–1984*, Gros, F. (ed.). Translated from the French by G. Burchell. New York: Palgrave Macmillan.

———.. (2013) *Lectures on the Will to Know: Lectures at the Collège de France 1970–1971*, D. Defert, (ed.). Translated from the French by G. Burchell. Basingstoke: Palgrave Macmillan.

———.. (2015) *The Punitive Society: Lectures at the Collège de France 1972–1973*, Harcourt, B., Ewald, F., Fontana, A., & Davidson, A. (eds.). Translated from the French by G. Burchell. Basingstoke: Palgrave Macmillan.

Fraser, N. (1989) *Unruly Practices: Power, Discourse, and Gender in Contemporary Social Theory*. Minneapolis: University of Minnesota Press.

Freud, S. (1937) "Analysis Terminable and Interminable", in Strachey, A., & Tyson, A. (eds.) *Moses and Monotheism: An Outline of Psycho-Analysis and Other Works*. Translated from the German by J. Strachey. London: The Hogarth Press and the Institute of Psycho-Analysis, pp. 211–253.

———. (1955) *Beyond the Pleasure Principle*, in *Sigmund Freud, The Standard Edition of the Complete Psychological Works of Sigmund Freud*. Edited and translated from the German by J. Strachey, A. Freud, A. Strachey, & Alan Tyson. London: The Hogarth Press.

———.(1963) "General Remarks on Hysterical Attacks (1909)", in Freud, S., & Rieff, P. (eds.) *Dora: An Analysis of a Case of Hysteria*. New York: Collier, pp. 123–124.

Ghamari-Tabrizi, B. (2016) *Foucault in Iran: Islamic Revolution after the Enlightenment*. Minneapolis: University of Minnesota Press.

Gildersleeve, M. (2016) "Method in the Madness: Hysteria and the Will to Power", *Social Sciences*, 5 (3), pp. 1–25.

Gotman, K. (2020) "Foucault, Oedipus, Négritude", in Fisher, T., & Gotman, K. (eds.) *Foucault's Theatres*. Manchester: Manchester University Press, pp. 63–81.

Grigg, R. (2008) *Lacan, Language, and Philosophy*. New York: SUNY Press.

Grigg, R., & Clemens, J. (eds.) (2006) *Jacques Lacan and the Other Side of Psychoanalysis: Reflections on Seminar XVII*. Durham: Duke University Press.

Gutting, G. (2003) "Review of Beatrice Han, Foucault's Critical Project", *Notre Dame Philosophical Reviews*, 5. Available at: https://philpapers.org/rec/GUTROB [Accessed: 20 January 2020].

———. (2005) *Foucault: A Very Short Introduction*. Oxford: Oxford University Press.

Habermas, J. (1987) *The Philosophical Discourse of Modernity: Twelve Lectures*. Translated from the German by F. G. Lawrence. Cambridge: The MIT Press.

———. (1989) "Taking Aim at the Heart of the Present: On Foucault's Lecture on Kant's What is Enlightenment?", in J. Habermas, *The New Conservatism: Cultural Criticism and the Historical Debate*, Edited & Translated from the German by S. W. Nicholsen. Cambridge: The MIT Press.

Han, B. (2002) *Foucault's Critical Project: Between the Transcendental and the Historical*. Stanford: Stanford University Press.

———. (2005) *The Analytic of Finitude and the History of Subjectivity*. Translated from the German by E. Pile, *The Cambridge Companion to Foucault*. Cambridge: Cambridge University Press, pp. 176–209.

———. (2010) "Death of Man': Foucault and Humanism", in Falzon, C. (ed.) *Foucault and Philosophy*. Oxford: Blackwell Publishing, pp. 118–142.

Hanssen, B. (2006) "Critical Theory and Poststructuralism: Foucault and Habermas", in Rush, F. (ed.) *The Cambridge Companion to Critical Theory*. Cambridge: Cambridge University Press, pp. 280– 309.

Haute, P. H. (2016) "Lacan Meets Freud? Patho-Analytic Reflections on the Status of the Perversions in Lacanian Metapsychology, *Studies in Gender and Sexuality*,17 (4), pp. 274–284.

Hayman, R. (1980) *Nietzsche: A Critical Life*. London: Willmer Brothers.

Hendricks, C. (2008) "Foucault's Kantian Critique: Philosophy and the Present", *Philosophy and Social Criticism*, 34, pp. 357–382.

Hendrix, J. S. (2019) "Jacques Lacan and Language", *Architecture, Art, and Historic Preservation*, Faculty Publications, 44.

Hoens, D. (2006) "Toward a New Perversion: Psychoanalysis", in Grigg, R., & Clemens, J. (eds.) *Jacques Lacan and the Other Side of Psychoanalysis: Reflections on Seminar XVII*. Durham: Duke University Press, pp. 88–104.

Hook, D. (2005) "Genealogy, Discourse, 'Effective History': Foucault and the Work of Critique", *Qualitative Research in Psychology*, 2 (1), pp. 3–31. https://doi.org/10.1191/1478088705qp025oa. [Accessed: 12 February 2020].

———. (2010) "The Powers of Emptiness", *Theory & Psychology*, 20 (6), pp. 855–870. Available at: https://doi.org/10.1177/0959354310383912 [Accessed: 22 January 2022].

———. (2013) "Nixon's 'full-speech': Imaginary and Symbolic Registers of Communication", *Journal of Theoretical and Philosophical Psychology*, 33 (1), pp. 32–50.

Houtman, C. (2003) "Lacan's Theory of the Four Discourses and The Sixth Sense", *Journal for Cultural Research*, 7 (3), pp. 277–296.

Huffer, L. (2020) *Foucault's Strange Eros*. New York: Columbia University Press.

Hyldgaard, K. (2004) "The Conformity of Perversion", *Symptom - Journal for Lacan*, 5.

Jose, J. (1998) *Biopolitics of the Subject: An Introduction to the Ideas of Michel Foucault*. Darwin: Northern Territory University Press.

Julien, P. (1994) *Jacques Lacan's Return to Freud the Real, the Symbolic and the Imaginary*. New York and London: New York University Press.

Kendall, G., & Wickham, G. (1999) *Using Foucault's Methods*. London: Sage.

Koopman, C. (*2010*) "Historical Critique or Transcendental Critique in Foucault: Two Kantian Lineages", *Foucault Studies*, 8, pp. 100–121.

———. (2013) *Genealogy as Critique: Foucault and the problems of modernity*. Bloomington: Indiana University Press.

Lacan, J. (1966) "Kant avec Sade" *in Écrits*. Paris: Editions du Seuil, pp. 763–92.

———. (1975) Introduction à l'édition allemande d'un premier volume des Écrits. *Scilicet*, 5, Paris: Éditions du Seuil.

———. (1977) "The Subversion of the Subject and the Dialectic of Desire in the Freudian Unconscious". Translated from the French by A. Sheridan, in *Écrits: A Selection*. London/New York: W.W. Norton and Company, pp. 292–325.

———. (1978) *The Seminar of Jacques Lacan, Book XI: The Four Fundamental Concepts of Psychoanalysis*, J. A. Miller (ed.). Translated from the French by A. Sheridan. New York/London: W. W. Norton & Company.

———. (1988a) *The Seminar of Jacques Lacan, Book I: Freud's Papers on Technique, 1953–1954*, J. A. Miller (ed.). Translated from the French by J. Forrester. Cambridge: Cambridge University Press.

———. (1988b) *The Seminar of Jacques Lacan, Book II. The Ego in Freud's Theory and in the Technique of Psychoanalysis, 1954–1955*, Miller, J. A. (ed.). Translated from the French by S. Tomaselli. New York: W. W. Norton & Company.

———. (1990) *Television: A Challenge to the Psychoanalytic Establishment*, J. Copjec (ed.). Translated from the French by D. Hollier. New York/London: W. W. Norton & Company.

———. (1992) *The Seminar of Jacques Lacan*, Book VII: The Ethics of Psychoanalysis, J. A. Miller (ed.). Translated from the French by D. Porter. New York/London: W.W. Norton & Company.

———. (1993) *The Seminar of Jacques Lacan, Book III: The Psychoses, 1955–1956*, J. A. Miller (ed.). Translated from the French by R. Grigg. New York/London: W. W. Norton & Company.

———. (1995) "The Position of the Unconscious", in R. Feldstein, B. Fink, & M. Jaanus (eds.) *Reading Seminar XI: Lacan's Four Fundamental Concepts of Psychoanalysis*. Translated from the French by B. Fink. Albany: SUNY Press, pp. 259–277.

———. (1998) *The Seminar XX, Encore: On Feminine Sexuality, the Limits of Love and Knowledge*, Miller, J. A. (ed.). Translated from the French by B. Fink. New York: W. W. Norton & Company.

———. (2001) *Écrits: A Selection*. Translated from the French by A. Sheridan. London: Routledge.

———. (2002) *Écrits*. Translated from the French by B. Fink, in collaboration with H. Fink & R. Grigg. New York: W.W. Norton.

———. (2007) *The Seminar of Jacques Lacan, Book XVII: The Other Side of Psychoanalysis, 1969–1970,* Miller, J. A. (ed.). Translated from the French by R. Grigg. New York: W.W. Norton and Company.

———. (2008) *My Teaching*, Miller, J. A (ed.). Translated from the French by D. Macey. London: Verso.

———. (2015) *The Seminar, Book VIII. Transference*, Miller, J. A. (ed.). Translated from the French by B. Fink. Cambridge: Polity.

Laclau, E. (2000) "Identity and Hegemony: The Role of Universality in the Constitution of Political Logics", in Butler, J. P. Laclau, E., & Zizek, S. (Eds.) *Contingency, Hegemony, Universality: Contemporary Dialogues on the Left*. London: Verso, pp. 44–89.

Laclau, E., & Mouffe, C. (1985) *Hegemony and Socialist Strategy: Towards a Radical Democratic Politics*. London: Verso.

Laclau, E., & Zac, L. (1994). "Minding the Gap: The Subject of Politics", in Laclau, E. (ed.) *The Making of Political Identities*. London/New York: Verso, pp. 11–39.

Lankshear, C. (2003). *Futures of Critical Theory: Dreams of Difference*. Oxford: Rowman & Littlefield Publishers.

Laurent, E. (2004) "Guiding Principles for Any Psychoanalytic Act". Available at: https://www.lacan.com/ericlaurent.html [Accessed: 22 January 2022].

Lawlor, L., & Nale, J. (eds.) (2020) *The Cambridge Foucault Lexicon*. Cambridge: United Kingdom Cambridge University Press.

Lazzarato, M. (2002) "From Biopower to Biopolitics", *Pli,* 13, pp. 99–113.

Leeb, C. (2020) "The Hysteric Rebels: Rethinking Radical Socio-Political Transformation with Foucault and Lacan", *Theory & Event,* 23 (3), pp. 607–640.

Luxon, N. (1994) "Truthfulness, Risk, and Trust in the Late Lectures of Michel Foucault", *Inquiry: An Interdisciplinary Journal of Philosophy,* 47 (5), pp. 464–489.

Maccannell, J. F. (2006) "More Thoughts for the Times on War and Death: The Discourse of Capitalism in Seminar XVII", in Grigg, R., & Clemens, J. (eds.) *Jacques Lacan and the Other Side of Psychoanalysis: Reflections on Seminar XVII*. Durham: Duke University Press, pp. 195–215.

Macey, D. (1988) *Lacan in contexts*. London: Verso.

———. (2005) *Michel Foucault.* London: Reaktion Books.

———. (2019) *The Lives of Michel Foucault: a Biography*. London: Verso.

Mahon, M. (1992) *Foucault's Nietzschean Genealogy: Truth, Power, and the Subject*. Albany: State University of New York Press.

Mahony, P. J. (2001) *Psychoanalysis and Discourse*. London: Brunner-Routledge.

Major-Poetzl, P. (1983) *Michel Foucault's Archaeology of Western Culture: Toward a New Science of History*. Chapel Hill: University of North Carolina Press.

Marx, K. (1951). *Theories of Surplus Value: a selection from the volumes published between 1905 to 1910 as Theorien uber den Mehrwert,* Kautsky, K. (ed.). London: Lawrence & Wishart.

———. (2019) *Capital: a Critique of Political Economy*. Oxford: Benediction Classics.

May, T. (2006) *The Philosophy of Foucault.* London: Acumen.

Mccarthy, T. (1990) "The Critique of Impure Reason: Foucault and the Frankfurt School", *Political Theory,* 18 (3), pp. 437–69. Available at: http://www.jstor.org/stable/191596. [Accessed: 12 February 2020].

Mcgushin, E. (2007) *Foucault's Askesis: An Introduction to the Philosophical Life*. Evanston: Northwestern University Press.

Mchoul, A W, & Grace, W. (1993) *A Foucault Primer: Discourse, Power and the Subject.* Melbourne: Melbourne University Press.

Mcnay, L. (1994) *Foucault: A Critical Introduction.* Cambridge: Polity Press.

Mcwhorter, L. (1999) *Bodies and Pleasures: Foucault and the Politics of Sexual Normalization*. Bloomington: Indiana University Press.

Mehlman, J. (1972) "The 'Floating Signifier': From Lévi-Strauss to Lacan", *Yale French Studies*, 48, pp. 10–37.

Mellard, J. M. (1991) *Using Lacan, Reading Fiction*. Urbana: University of Illinois Press.

Merquior, J. G. (1985) *Foucault*. London: Fontana.

Micale, M. S. (2019) *Approaching Hysteria: Disease and its Interpretations*. New Jersey: Princeton University Press.

Miller, J.-A. (2000) "Paradigms of Jouissance", *Lacanian Ink,* 17, pp. *10–47.*

———. (1996) "On perversion", in Feldstein, R., Fink, B., & Jaanus, M. (eds.) *Reading Seminars I and II: Lacan's Return to Freud*. Albany: SUNY, pp. 306–320.

Milner, J. C. (2021) A Search for Clarity: Science and Philosophy in Lacan's Oeuvre. Translated from the French by E. Pluth. Northwestern University Press.

Mitchell, J., *&* Rose, J. (eds.) (*1982) Feminine Sexuality*. Jacques Lacan and the École *Freudienne*. London: Macmillan Press Ltd

Moi, T. (1985) "Representation of Patriarchy: Sexuality and Epistemology in Freud's Dora", in Bernheimer, C., & Kahane, C. (eds.) *Dora's Case Freud–Hysteria–Feminism*. West Sussex: Columbia University Press, pp. 181–199.

Moretti, A. (2021) "Agonistic Truth: The Issue of Power Between the Will to Knowledge and Government by Truth", in Faustino, M. & Ferraro, G. (eds.) *The Late Foucault: Ethical and Political Questions*. London: Bloomsbury Academic, pp. 133–148.

Moroncini, B. (2009) "On Love. Jacques Lacan and Plato's Symposium" *European Journal of Psychoanalysis*, 25. Available at: https://www.journal-psychoanalysis.eu/on-love-jacques-lacan-and-platos-symposium/ [Accessed: 22 January 2022].

Nancy, J. C., & Lacoue-Labarthe, P. (1992) *The Title of the Letter: A Reading of Lacan*. Translated from the French by F. Raffoul & D. Pettigrew. Albany: State University of New York Press.

Nietzsche (2007) On the Genealogy of Morality, in Ansell-Pearson, K. (ed.) *Cambridge Texts in the History of Political Thought*. Cambridge: Cambridge University Press.

——— (1968) *The Will to Power*. Translated from the German by R. J. Hollingdale and W. A. Kaufmann. New York: Vintage Books.

Nobus, D. (2000) *Jacques Lacan and the Freudian Practice of Psychoanalysis*. New York: Routledge.

———. (1998) *Key Concepts of Lacanian Psychoanalysis*. New York: Other Press.

O'Farrell, C. (1989) *Foucault: Historian or Philosopher?* London: Macmillan.

———. (2005) *Michel Foucault.* London: Sage Publications.

O'leary, T. (2002) *Foucault and the Art of Ethics*. London: Continuum.

Olssen, M. (2003) "Foucault and Critique: Kant, Humanism and the Human Sciences", in Peters, M. A., Olssen, M., & Lankshear, C. (eds.) *Futures of Critical Theory*. New York: Rowman & Littlefield, pp. 73–102.

Peters, M., & Appel, S. (1996) "Positioning Theory: Discourse, The Subject and the Problem of Desire", *Social Analysis*, 40, pp. 120–141. Available at: http://www.jstor.org/stable/23171700 [Accessed: 12 February 2020].

Prado, C. G. (1995) *Starting with Foucault: An Introduction to Genealogy.* Boulder: Westview Press.

Rabinow, P. (ed.) (1984) *The Foucault Reader*. New York: Pantheon Books.

Ragland, E. (2006) "The Hysteric's Truth", in Grigg, R., & Clemens, J. (eds.) *Jacques Lacan and the Other Side of Psychoanalysis: Reflections on Seminar XVII*. Durham: Duke University Press, pp. 69–87.

Ragland-Sullivan, E. (1987) *Jacques Lacan and the Philosophy of Psychoanalysis.* Urbana/Chicago: University of Illinois Press.

Rajchman, J. (1985) *Michel Foucault: The Freedom of Philosophy*. New York: Columbia University Press.

———. (1986) "Lacan and the Ethics of Modernity", *Representations*, 15, pp. 42–56.

———. (1988) "Habermas's Complaint", *New German Critique*, 45, pp. 163–191.

———. (1991) *Truth and Eros: Foucault, Lacan and the Question of Ethics.* New York/London: Routledge.

Raulet, G. (1983) "Structuralism and Post-Structuralism: An Interview with Michel Foucault", *Télos*, 55, pp. 195-211.

Read, J. (2009) "A Genealogy of Homo-Economicus: Neoliberalism and the Production of Subjectivity", *Foucault Studies*, 6, pp. 25–36.

Rocco, C. (1997) *Tragedy and Enlightenment: Athenian Political Thought and the Dilemmas of Modernity.* Berkeley: University of California Press.

Rorty, R. (1986) "Foucault and Epistemology", in Hoy, D. C. (ed.) *Foucault: A Critical Reader*. Oxford: Basil Blackwell, pp. 41–50.

Rose, J. (1985) "Dora: Fragment of an Analysis", in Bernheimer, C., & Kahane, C. (eds.) *Dora's Case Freud–Hysteria–Feminism*. West Sussex: Columbia University Press, pp. 128–148.

Roudinesco, E. (1990), *Jacques Lacan & Co.: A History of Psychoanalysis in France, 1925–1985*. Translated from the French by J. Mehlman. Chicago: University of Chicago Press.

Rouse, J. (2005) "Power/Knowledge", in Gutting, G. (ed.) *The Cambridge Companion to Foucault*. Cambridge: Cambridge University Press, pp. 95–122.

Salecl, R. (1998) *(Per)versions of love and hate*. London: Verso.

Schmidt, J., & Wartenberg, T. E. (1994) "Foucault's Enlightenment: Critique, Revolution, and the Fashioning of the Self", in Kelly, M. (ed.) *Critique and Power: Recasting the Foucault/Habermas Debate*. Cambridge: MIT Press.

Schmidt, J. (2013) *"On Foucault's Review of Cassirer's Philosophy* of the Enlightenment", *Persistent Enlightenment*. Available at: http://persistentenlightenment.wordpress.com/2013/07/02/foucaultcassirer/. [Accessed: 27 January 2021].

Schroeder, J. L. (2008) *The Four Lacanian Discourses: or Turning Law Inside-out*. London: Birbeck Law.

Scott, C. E. (1990) *The Question of Ethics: Nietzsche, Foucault, Heidegger*. Bloomington: Indiana University.

Sheridan, A. (1980) *Michel Foucault: The Will to Truth*. London: Tavistock Publications.

———. (2015) *Michel Foucault: The Will to Truth*. Abingdon, OX: Routledge.

Soler, C. (1996) "The Symbolic Order (I)", in Feldstein, R., Fink, B., & Jaanus M. (eds.) *Reading Seminars I & II Lacan's return to Freud*. New Jersey: SUNY Press: pp. 39–46.

———. (2019) *Lacan: The Unconscious Reinvented*. London: Routledge.

Swales, S. (2012) *Perversion: A Lacanian Psychoanalytic Approach to the Subject*. New York: Routledge.

Tarpey, T. (2011) "Lacan's Psychoanalytic Way of Love". Available at: https://lacancircle.com.au/psychoanalysislacan-journal/psychoanalysislacan-volume-1/lacans-psychoanalytic-way-of-love/ [Accessed: 22 January 2022].

Taylor, D., & Vintges, K. (2004) *Feminism and the Final Foucault*. Urbana, IL: University of Illinois Press.

Thompson, K. (2008) "Historicity and Transcendentality: Foucault, Cavaillès, and the Phenomenology of the Concept", *History and Theory*, 47 (1), pp. 1–18.

Tomšič, S. (2015) *The Capitalist Unconscious: Marx and Lacan*. London: Verso.

Torfing, J. (1999) *New Theories of Discourse: Laclau, Mouffe, and Zizek*. Oxford: Blackwell Publishers.

Van Haute, P., & Geyskens, T. (2016) "Freud's Dream? Lacan and Oedipus", in TomŠiČ, S., & Zevnik, A. (eds.), *Jacques Lacan between Psychoanalysis and Politics*. London/New York: Routledge, pp. 47–61.

Verhaeghe, P. (*1999*) *Does* the *Woman Exist*? From *Freud's Hysteric* to *Lacan's Feminine*. Translated from the French by *M. D. RY.* New York: Other Press.

———. (2006) "Enjoyment and Impossibility: Lacan's Revision of the Oedipus Complex", in Grigg, R., & Clemens, J. (eds.) *Jacques Lacan and the Other Side of Psychoanalysis: Reflections on Seminar XVII*. Durham: Duke University Press, pp. 29–50.

Vernant, J.-P., Vidal-Naquet, P., & Lloyd, J. (1990) *Myth and Tragedy in Ancient Greece*. New York: Zone Books.

Viltard, M. (1999) "Foucault, Lacan: La Leçon Des Ménines", *L'Unebévue*, 12, pp. 57–90.

Wajcman, G. (2003) "The Hysteric's Discourse", in ŽiŽek, S. (ed.) *Jacques Lacan: Critical Evaluations in Cultural Theory*. Vol 1: Psychoanalytic Theory and Practice. New York: Routledge, pp. 186–198.

Wright, C. (2016) "Discourse and the Master's Lining: A Lacanian Critique of the Globalizing (Bio)Politics of the Diagnostic and Statistical Manual", in Tomšič, S., & Zevnik, A. (eds.), *Jacques Lacan: between Psychoanalysis and Politics*. London: Routledge.

Žižek, S. (1989) *The Sublime Object of Ideology*. London & New York: Verso.

———. (1992) *Looking Awry: An Introduction to Jacques Lacan through Popular Culture*. Cambridge: MIT Press.

———. (1998) "Four Discourses, Four Subjects", in Žižek, S. (ed.) *Cogito and the Unconscious*. Durham: University of Duke Press, pp. 74–113.

———. (2000) "Class Struggle or Postmodernism? Yes, please!", in Butler, J., Laclau, E., & Žižek, S. (eds.) *Contingency, Hegemony, Universality*. London: Verso, pp. 90–135.

———. (2009) *The Ticklish Subject: The Absent Centre of Political Ontology*. London: Verso.

———. (2016) "Can One Exit From the Capitalist Discourse Without Becoming a Saint", *Crisis and Critique*, 3 (3). Available at: http://crisiscritique.org/political11/Slavoj.pdf. [Accessed: 27 January 2021].

Zupančič, A.(2000) *The Ethics of the Real: Kant and Lacan*. London/New York: Verso.

———. (2006) "When Surplus Enjoyment Meets Surplus Value", in Grigg, R., & Clemens, J. (eds.) *Jacques Lacan and the Other Side of Psychoanalysis: Reflections on Seminar XVII*. Durham: Duke University Press, pp. 155–178.

———. (2016) "Biopolitics, Sexuality and the Unconscious". Paragraph, 39(1), 49–64.

Index[1]

[1] Note: Page numbers followed by 'n' refer to notes.

J. L. Davis, *Reading Foucault Through Lacan*, The Palgrave Lacan Series,
https://doi.org/10.1007/978-3-031-69738-8

GPSR Compliance
The European Union's (EU) General Product Safety Regulation (GPSR) is a set of rules that requires consumer products to be safe and our obligations to ensure this.

If you have any concerns about our products, you can contact us on

ProductSafety@springernature.com

In case Publisher is established outside the EU, the EU authorized representative is:

Springer Nature Customer Service Center GmbH
Europaplatz 3
69115 Heidelberg, Germany

www.ingramcontent.com/pod-product-compliance
Lightning Source LLC
Chambersburg PA
CBHW071553310826
50743CB00004B/138
* 9 7 8 3 0 3 1 6 9 7 3 7 1 *